T0369368

Autism
Believe in the Future

From Infancy to Independence

Ann Millan

iUniverse, Inc.
New York Bloomington

Autism–Believe in the Future
From Infancy to Independence

iUniverse books may be ordered through booksellers or by contacting:

iUniverse
1663 Liberty Drive
Bloomington, IN 47403
www.iuniverse.com
1-800-Authors (1-800-288-4677)

Because of the dynamic nature of the Internet, any Web addresses or links contained in this book may have changed since publication and may no longer be valid. The views expressed in this work are solely those of the author and do not necessarily reflect the views of the publisher, and the publisher hereby disclaims any responsibility for them.

ISBN: 978-1-4502-2184-9 (pbk)
ISBN: 978-1-4502-2186-3 (cloth)
ISBN: 978-1-4502-2185-6 (ebook)

Printed in the United States of America

iUniverse rev. date: 6/21/10

Contents

Dedication

In memory of Roger, who had classic autism and died in 2007 at thirty-two years of age.
Roger was on a cocktail of psychotropic and prescription drugs and lived in an excellent group home. His death certificate lists cause of death as combined drug toxicity.

and

Thank you to the late Senator Edward M. Kennedy, for your significant part in all the legislation that has benefited individuals with disabilities.

Acknowledgments

Thank you, Robin, for allowing me to tell your story. I know that some subjects are sensitive and bring back memories you'd rather forget; however, your courage in helping other people learn about autism is a testimony to your success.

Many people have touched our lives, providing Robin with encouragement and support throughout the years. They have definitely influenced who she is today. Looking back, it is amazing how we found *quality* therapists and other professionals who had expertise working with autism almost forty years ago. They all helped draw Robin's roadmap for success, and I hope I have acknowledged their critical roles in her development throughout this book.

Bob, my husband, has been my major book reviewer. Rewrite after rewrite, we have relived Robin's journey with autism, amazed at her continued achievements over the years. For Robin's sisters, Pam and Karen, their contributions made this book possible. We were able to discuss our family dynamics–some for the first time–which brought us all closer with better understanding.

A special thank you to LorRainne Jones, MA, CCC-SLP, PhD, and director of Kid Pro Therapy Services, Inc., Tampa, Florida, and to Tina Phillips, president and CEO of Palm Beach Habilitation Center.

In addition, extra credit belongs to friends, caregivers, professionals, and even some strangers who came to my rescue with encouragement and suggestions to help me highlight Robin's significant milestones: Zeena Zeidberg, MA; Filomena Macdonald; Leah Pradee, PT; Beverley DeStories; Elaine LeFebvre; Judy Koehn; Michelle Eline; Patty Houghland; Kitty Baugh; Richard Wolkind; Kathleen Tehrani; Nancy Cale; Clinton Kent; Reem Tarantino; and Olivia Macdonald.

Most important, our family's faith in God has kept us on track for Robin. Without it, she would not be where she is today. Thank you, Lord.

Foreword

In *Autism—Believe in the Future*, Ann Millan provides an inspiring and wonderfully written story about overcoming the odds. In 1971, when Ann's daughter, Robin, was born, autism was still a rare disorder. At that time, most children diagnosed with autism were placed in residential facilities. In the mid-1970s, when mandatory public school programs became available, Ann was very excited, but that excitement soon turned to disappointment as she realized that early specialized education services for children with severe disabilities were often inadequate. Too often, educators, who were providing the services for the first time, had no idea how to effectively educate such children. In spite of disappointments and overwhelming odds, Ann never gave up her fight against the disabilities that were taking her daughter. Despite the odds against them, she was determined to find a way to help Robin.

Early on, many professionals that Ann sought out did not offer hope, let alone suggestions or recommendations for how to help Robin overcome her deficits and learn the skills she would need to become independent. The education and therapy opportunities that they provided to Robin were not appropriate and did not address her needs. Robin's difficulty and lack of success was not, Ann argued, "due to her deficits." Rather, she felt, the difficulties were the result of intervention that did not suit Robin's learning style. Sometimes improvements seen in the home were not seen in school. For example, after reading popular magazines of the day, Ann decided to put Robin on the Feingold diet. Her family saw positive behavioral changes at home. But sadly, in the school and therapy settings, no changes in behavior were reported.

Not to be outdone and refusing to give up, Ann persisted. Along the way she was able to find "strategic" professionals, who provided insight and recommendations for interventions that were right for Robin at a given point in time. One such professional was a speech therapist who worked closely with Ann, providing effective behavior management strategies. With the change in diet and the behavioral strategies, Ann felt Robin was ready for learning.

As her discouragement with the educational programs mounted, Ann, with no training as a teacher or therapist, decided it was time to take the ball into her own hands. First, she had to figure out exactly how Robin learned—

not an easy task. Second, she had to identify the most effective methodology and materials for teaching Robin. The third step was to set up an appropriate educational program for Robin. This task was the easy part—and the hard part. Easy because Ann would no longer be wasting precious time and energy trying to explain how to teach Robin to others. Hard because Ann would be on her own as the primary instructor. With determination and strong family support, she embraced the work before her—hour after hour, day after day, month after month, year after year.

Autism—Believe in the Future is the story of how Ann did it. It is an interesting and compelling read—not unlike a mystery novel—in which the author must collect clues and figure out the mystery of how to teach her daughter. As an infant, Robin had a severe reaction to her immunizations and was diagnosed as extremely colicky. As a toddler, she was non-verbal, extremely reactive to sensory stimuli, severely withdrawn, and she displayed challenging behaviors. A diagnosis of "mentally retarded and emotionally disturbed" was given. Because her disability was so severe, Robin's prognosis was poor at best. But prognosticators can be wrong. Today, at age thirty-eight, Robin lives independently in her own condominium, has her own car (a PT Cruiser), lightens her hair to just the right shade of blonde, tries to be a "hipper" dresser than her mom (no dowdy clothes for her), holds two jobs, and has a boyfriend. Ann provides a detailed analysis of each step along the way. From early diagnosis to independence, it is an incredible journey.

Ann's story sends many important and timely messages to parents. First and foremost is the message of hope. This message of hope comes with a caveat. It is critical that the program developed for each child fit the child—not merely the diagnosis of autism. The intervention must combine the right pieces to accommodate how the child learns. Many children diagnosed with severe autism can make significant gains and achieve some level of independence. Secondly, Ann provides a message of empowerment. Parents must feel that, with support, they can help their child acquire the skills necessary for independence. The third message of hope is that even as a child grows into adulthood, he or she can continue to learn new skills and increase their independence.

Also impressive is that Ann achieved so much without the benefit of the popular "gold standard" autism intervention protocol: thirty to forty hours a week of one-on-one instruction provided by individuals trained in applied behavior analysis (ABA). Such a program can be cost prohibitive, a cost paid by families, insurance companies, and/or the education dollars in states where an intensive ABA approach is funded. While ABA is certainly an evidence-based intervention for children with autism, parent-provided instruction or intervention, such as Robin's, under the direction of a person with expertise in a particular type of intervention, is gaining acceptance.[1]

I first met Robin when she was twenty-eight years old. She had just started the Defeat Autism Now (DAN) protocol for diet and vitamin supplements. Ann was excited about Robin's improvements since starting DAN. She initially contacted me to get information about Fast ForWord, a computer-based program designed to improve language and reading skills. Ann hoped that improvements in these skills would make it easier for Robin to find a job in an office setting, which was Robin's dream.

My first step was to get Robin started with Interactive Metronome Therapy (IM) to improve her speed and accuracy of processing auditory information. This would help improve Robin's processing and conversation skills. Subsequently, Robin participated in other auditory-based intervention programs, including Fast ForWord from Scientific Learning Corporation and Rhythmic Entrainment Intervention (REI).[2]

Most recently, Robin and her parents have initiated Relationship Development Intervention (RDI). How exciting that has been! Robin has shown steady and impressive gains. She has learned to communicate with more than words; she now expertly "reads" facial expressions, body language, gestures, and vocal emphasis. Ann has made impressive gains as well. She has learned to slow down and be less imperative and more declarative in her communication. Ann is learning, slowly and systematically, to "step back" and allow Robin to "step forward"—competently embracing life in the dynamic and ever-changing world in which we live.

I am excited to be a part of Robin's continued growth as she becomes a more confident and happy adult who happens to have autism. There is no doubt that Ann was a trailblazer. Her accomplishments suggest that her vision for Robin is becoming reality. In this book, Ann shares her story with other parents so that they will have hope and will feel empowered. She wants parents to know that it is possible to beat the odds and believe in the future!

LorRainne Jones, MA, CCC-SLP, PhD
Director, Kid Pro Therapy Services, Inc.
Tampa, Florida

---

1   DIR/Floortime model (www.floortime.org); Hanen, More Than Words (www.hanen.org); Rethink Autism (www.rethinkautism.com).

2   Interactive Metronome Therapy (IM) (www.interactivemetronome.com); Rhythmic Entrainment Intervention (REI) (www.reiinstitute.com); Relationship Development Intervention (RDI) (www.rdiconnect.com); Fast ForWord from Scientific Learning Corporation (www.scilearn.com).

Preface

Individuals living with autism deserve the opportunity to become productive adults, a part of their community, and employed. Professionals must understand that *all* individuals with autism have incredible potential. They must support families, limit their own judgments, and appreciate each family's dynamics.

Bob and I have three girls. The third, Robin, has *classic* autism. For years, we felt Robin's future was at the mercy of professionals. As they continually discouraged us, we were just as determined not to allow them to crush our dreams for her, even though we couldn't visualize her future. We loved her and felt she should have the same opportunities as our other children. As months turned into years, we were overwhelmed with her disabilities: behavior, chemical sensitivity, speech and language, social, and mental (a diagnosis of mental retardation was given). This is a lot! Where would we start?

It wasn't easy. Autism intervention required our personal commitment. For Robin, *everything* she learned had to be tailored to her unique learning style—*every time*. She didn't need just *one* thing or *one* therapy to reach her independence. Robin needed them all and she needed them all in a coordinated manner.

Despite Robin's obvious disabilities, we did not allow ourselves to make excuses. Today, many states have massive waiting lists for services, inadequate services, or no services at all. Many school systems still cannot meet the needs of individuals with autism. However, when you make excuses like "I'm on a waiting list" or "It's not available" or "I don't know where to start," you're wasting your child's precious time.

Bob and I certainly are not the only parents who succeeded in overcoming autism for their child in adulthood, but we are definitely among the few. I now realize that, just like any other health condition, like diabetes or high blood pressure, stabilization for Robin's autism is life long. Today, Robin's biomedical interventions and language therapy are her stabilizers, allowing her to remain employed and live independently in the community. I much prefer this lifestyle for her, rather than the alternative of a cocktail of prescription drugs, physical restraints, or institutional placement.

I hope the reader will benefit from our family's autism roadmap. My goal is to encourage every parent to expect *at least* the same results for their child—and it doesn't need to take them thirty-eight years to do it. The key for parents is to empower themselves to recognize *quality* supports, priorities, shortcuts, and gaps needing to be addressed.

I'm not a superhero, just a regular mom with a lot of determination. I draw my strength from my faith, my strong upbringing, and the lessons of my art teacher in the seventh grade, Mrs. Lovejoy. She never allowed us to use the word *can't*—and I never allowed myself to use the word *can't* with Robin!

How to Read This Book

Robin's unique needs and learning style are addressed in specific chapters to show readers the importance of each intervention for autism. They can be read separate of each other; however, the full impact of Robin's autism journey is interrelated and can only be truly appreciated as a whole.

Definition of Autism

Centers for Disease Control and Prevention (CDC)

Autism spectrum disorders (ASDs) are a group of developmental disabilities caused by a problem with the brain. Scientists do not know yet exactly what causes this problem. ASDs can impact a person's functioning at different levels, from very mildly to severely. There is usually nothing about how a person with an ASD looks that sets them apart from other people, but they may communicate, interact, behave, and learn in ways that are different from most people. The thinking and learning abilities of people with ASDs can vary—from gifted to severely challenged. Autistic disorder is the most commonly known type of ASD, but there are others, including "pervasive developmental disorder—not otherwise specified" (PDD-NOS) and Asperger syndrome.

- *Autistic Disorder* (also called "classic" autism) This is what most people think of when hearing the word "autism." People with autistic disorder usually have significant language delays, social and communication challenges, and unusual behaviors and interests. Many people with autistic disorder also have intellectual disability.
- *Asperger Syndrome* People with Asperger syndrome usually have some milder symptoms of autistic disorder. They might have social challenges and unusual behaviors and interests. However, they typically do not have problems with language or intellectual disability.
- *Pervasive Developmental Disorder—Not Otherwise Specified* (PDD-NOS; also called "atypical autism") People who meet some of the criteria for autistic disorder or Asperger syndrome, but not all, may be diagnosed with PDD-NOS. People with PDD-NOS usually have fewer and milder symptoms than those with autistic disorder. The symptoms might cause only social and communication challenges.

www.cdc.gov

PART I
Robin's Experience

You have only failed when you have failed to try

—Plaque over my kitchen sink

Chapter 1:
Robin's Journey in a Capsule

Infancy

Robin was born on April 26, 1971. Her Apgar, which evaluates a newborn's physical condition, was 10, the best score possible. She was our smallest child, weighing eight pounds. I had concerns during my pregnancy because this baby wasn't as active in my womb as her sisters, Pam and Karen. My gynecologist assured me everything was fine. After labor began, my doctor met me at the hospital, I checked in, and he returned to his downtown office. Once I started to crown, the nurse gave me the anesthesia epidural to slow down my baby's delivery until the doctor returned. Robin was dark purple when she was born. In 1971, fathers were not allowed in the delivery room. I did not know to request an on-call house doctor to help me.

Before Robin was born, I asked my general practitioner, Dr. Reed (not his real name), if he would also be Robin's medical doctor. I felt our pediatrician's office was too crowded and a maze of germs. He agreed. After Robin was born, Dr. Reed visited us in the hospital and assured me that everything was fine.

Robin's first month was such ecstasy. She was a perfect baby, almost too perfect. She slept most of the time and seldom cried. The girls were thrilled with their new sister. Both girls were in school, Karen in half-day kindergarten and Pam second grade. Life was good.

Everything quickly changed at the one-month mark, when Robin had her first appointment with Dr. Reed. He gave Robin her first Diphtheria, Pertussis, and Tetanus (DPT) shot. His medical chart notes read as follows:

"1 month check up, gained 2 ½ lbs. Doing fine & breast-feeding. No colic or bowel upset. No difficulty. DPT #1. Start cereal, fruit, vegetables."

When we arrived home from Robin's appointment, she was asleep in her car seat. As I picked her up to go inside, she startled and let out a wild high-pitched scream, as if she was in intense pain. Thinking I had accidently stuck her with an open diaper pin, I rushed into the house and stripped off her clothes. The diaper pins were fine. I tried everything to console her, but she continued the same wild, intense screaming for eight long hours. She didn't feel hot, so I didn't take her temperature. Then, as quickly as she started screaming, she sank into a deep sleep. I thought she was just exhausted. I know I was!

I was nursing and several feedings had passed. Each time I checked her diaper, it was dry, yet each time I tried to wake or touch her, she let out the same intense scream. I thought she just needed to sleep it off.

After Karen left for afternoon kindergarten the next day, I picked Robin up to nurse. She screamed as I moved her, then exploded with diarrhea. After that day, our lives changed forever! Robin was never the same child we had brought home from the hospital just one month before. Nine days later, Robin's bowels were not back to normal, she continued to be defensive to touch, and she continued screaming wildly all waking hours. I called Dr. Reed's office and the nurse sent out a prescription for colic. It didn't help.

I took Robin back to Dr. Reed for her second month checkup. The nurse was very concerned when she saw Robin. Dr. Reed came into the room.

"What did you do to my baby?" I said.

He assured me she was fine and gave Robin her second DPT shot, saying I had to complete the vaccine series once it was started. That afternoon, I called his office. I couldn't get Robin to sleep because of her wild screaming. Again, he said she had colic. A month later, Robin received her third DPT shot. This time, I changed doctors.

Before Robin's first appointment with Dr. Reed, she was an easy and content baby. She nursed and slept well for a one month old. She seldom cried, and we could hold her over our shoulder and on our lap. She didn't complain when we touched her or changed her clothes or diapers. The girls loved helping me give her a bath. She was beginning to follow us with her eyes when we moved around her. After Robin's one-month doctor's appointment, she lost all these basic skills, and after three months they still had not returned.

At three months old, Robin's eyes were permanently crossed. She couldn't hold her head up or even give a reactive smile. She wouldn't let any of us hold her in our arms to comfort her, including me. We couldn't hold her over our shoulder or on our lap. We did find we could hold her face-down toward the floor, holding her *firmly* on our forearm. In this position, the screaming was a little less intense.

Robin just needed stimulation, I thought. After our planned move to our new home, when she was three months old, I went into the mode of *fixing* her. I honestly believed she'd get over the reaction to the shot, just like a cold or an ear infection. Dr. Reed kept insisting that vaccines do not have reactions. I was confused and assumed she'd recover because she wasn't like this her first month.

I had four record albums that I would play every day, with the volume high enough for her to hear over her screaming. I played the same four albums repeatedly when she was awake. I danced around the house and sang to the music, holding her firmly and gently bouncing her on my forearm. My favorite songs were Helen Reddy's "I Am Woman," Simon and Garfunkel's "Bridge over Troubled Waters," Roger Miller's "King of the Road," and the Hillside Singers' "I'd Like to Teach the World to Sing (In Perfect Harmony)." (Having just typed these titles, I never before saw the humor in this selection!) My arm constantly ached.

Robin treated us all as if we were an intrusion into her world. There was no feeling of warmth as I'd had with the other girls. Oh, how I tried to get her to accept a pacifier or blanket for comfort. Because of the unexplainable changes in her behavior, I never started the doctor's recommended foods. I needed to understand what was wrong with Robin first. I was nursing, was it my milk? I was so careful about what I ate. I nursed lying on the bed—not touching her—so she could relax while eating. I stopped nursing her at five months old, hoping for a positive behavior change. *Maybe she was allergic to my milk.* None came.

I was concerned Robin was sleeping too much. She had her own bedroom and I usually had to wake her up to start the day or after naps. Many times her naps ran into each other, morning and afternoon. I was concerned that her delayed development might be the result of sleeping too much.

I requested another Phenylketonuria (PKU) test from Robin's new pediatrician, which I thought ruled out mental retardation. It was negative. He continued to assure me she was fine and she'd outgrow it.

At seven months old, Robin should have been rolling over and beginning to sit up, but she wasn't. I began to alternate our dancing to the music with floor exercises. I would roll her over while holding her head or pull her to a sitting position. I kept moving her body gently with my hands. I would rattle toys and sing to the music. I tried to get her to notice things around her, including me. But she did not see me—she seemed to look through me.

By ten months old, there was still no change in Robin. She didn't respond to doors slamming or to visual stimuli. Her body was like a ragdoll most of the time. Diaper changes, baths, eating, and car rides were always a battle, because they required us to touch her. We dreaded taking her anywhere.

Bob and I feared Robin might be blind and deaf. The girls were devastated and confused, and so was I.

One to Four Years Old

After Robin turned twelve months old, within a six-week period she held her head up, rolled over, sat up, crawled, climbed stairs, and stood at the coffee table, screaming all the while. She also added the fine art of biting her hand to her talents. Because of this, she developed a severe callus on her right thumb joint.

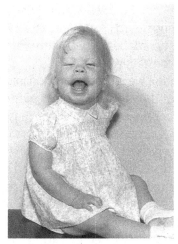

Fig. 1.1. Robin at fourteen months old.

I knew better than to think Robin had caught up in development. In fact, I was even more confused. This was her first growth *spurt* and we wanted more. We just didn't understand. Her mental development appeared to still be at the infancy level, even though her physical development appeared to be catching up with her age. She made no language sounds (like *da da*) and she still did not seem to see or hear anything around her. She didn't smile.

Robin's new pediatrician was not listening to me. Frustrated, I made an appointment with Dr. Reed. He was still my MD, and I didn't know what else to do. When he saw Robin this time, he too was very concerned. He referred us to the Birth Defects Clinic at the local Children's Hospital National Medical Center, Washington, D.C. Dr. Reed thought Robin might have Down's syndrome. I didn't agree with him, but I was relieved that finally somebody was listening to us—even if it was the doctor who diagnosed her as having colic!

As Robin continued to remain in her own little world of screaming and sleeping, we skipped from hospital to hospital looking for answers—Children's Hospital National Medical Center, Birth Defects Clinic; Georgetown University Hospital; George Washington University Hospital—no one had any answers. Robin was not a Down's syndrome child. We got *no* help or advice to deal with her screaming or her crossed eyes. They did not give us a diagnosis or a label.

Robin didn't regress after her original physical *spurt*, but she didn't progress either. I continued working with her during all waking hours, thinking it was important to keep her stimulated. At eighteen months old she took off running while screaming and biting her hand at the same time. She ran in a big circle through the kitchen, living room, dining room, and back through the kitchen, again and again and again. If I tried to stop her, she would literally fight to get away from me. Then, if I let her, she'd continue where she left off.

Obviously, Robin could *see* something—what we weren't quite sure. She wasn't bumping into walls, furniture, or people, but she easily tripped over her own two feet, resulting in trips to the emergency room. We still questioned her hearing.

When Robin was younger, I had become an expert at shifting from activity to activity during our floor exercises. Now that she liked to run, running had become a safety issue. I could not allow her to run uncontrollably all over the house. I substituted the inappropriate behavior (running) by dressing her in costumes—hats, scarves, shoes, jewelry, and so on. We provided a lot of variety. With these costumes, she was finally allowing us to touch her! After several years of this routine, I could almost feel her hesitate as we went to the costume box, perhaps anticipating our next move. She had access to the costume box, but it never occurred to her to play in it. Robin didn't play.

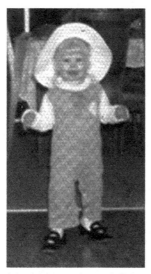

Fig. 1.2. Robin's costumes slowed down her running.

When I couldn't correct a behavior by changing the activity, *timeout* was my only option. A baby safety-gate across Robin's bedroom doorway provided a safe place for a timeout. I was afraid of emotional scars to shut her bedroom door. Robin spent a lot of time in timeout and she hated it, which actually was a good thing. At least she was showing emotion, I thought.

I was continually looking for ways to help Robin. She seemed so angry all the time and couldn't enjoy us as a family. Every day was an exhausting and overwhelming bad day for her, but some days were actually worse than others. We couldn't understand this behavior, which we called her "good day/bad day syndrome."

We continued with our semi-annual checkups at Children's Hospital National Medical Center, Birth Defects Clinic, seeking help for Robin. When she was two, they referred us to a local county social worker, who in turn referred us to Muriel Humphrey School for Retarded Children, supported by our local Association for Retarded Children (ARC). They evaluated Robin and accepted her into their school.

While Robin was at Muriel Humphrey, I finally found an opthamologist to correct her crossed eyes. He performed surgery and prescribed glasses for Robin. About the same time, Robin started the Feingold diet for hyperactivity in children. The Feingold diet focused on eliminating artificial preservatives and colorings from a person's diet (see chapter 2: Diet, Vitamins, and Supplements).

Robin attended Muriel Humphrey for two years and she liked the routine. She was in a class with all Down's syndrome children. Her teacher, El Peoples, potty trained her and said she was very stimulating to the class!

Robin made a lot of progress at Muriel Humphrey and her test scores dramatically improved. The school closed the following year because the public school system began providing special education services according to a new law (PL 94-142—Education of All Handicapped Children Act). The public school system was only offering *afternoon* classes for Robin's age group, and Muriel Humphrey's psychologist felt Robin's school routine of half-day morning classes should not be changed. Robin was still very dependent on her afternoon naps. Therefore, he recommended we place Robin in a regular private prekindergarten morning program.

Philip DeVore, Muriel Humphrey School Psychological Assessment, Robin 3 years old

"This mother has learned a great deal about the child. When the psychological examination was reviewed with her, and she sat in on the testing, it was evident that she is completely aware of Robin's abilities and deficits."

Philip DeVore, Muriel Humphrey School Psychological, Robin 4 years old

"Robin is a much changed child. The big change one sees is her speech. She has abundant speech. She does not use it appropriately always, but most of the time, she is right there responding to questions. It is evident the parents expect of her what they would expect of any of their other children. For instance, they are able to turn her loose in the neighborhood and she has the control to stay nearby."

After looking at several schools, we placed Robin in our church preschool program. They assured me they could handle her. Robin attended Mrs. Burgess's morning class twice a week for two months before they asked us to find another school placement for Robin. The diet made a big difference in Robin at home, but it was not enough to cope with the outside world. I requested Mrs. Burgess's justification in writing. With this letter in hand, we were finally able to push Robin's pediatrician for drug therapy.

Mrs. Burgess, Preschool Teacher, Robin 4 years old

"Robin is an extremely active child who smiles frequently and enjoys all the large muscle activities … She has a very short attention span … It is extremely hard to control her wandering and running from the classroom during her bad days, which are the majority … Her relationships with the other children range from parallel play on good days to disruption only on bad days … children are afraid of her because she frequently pushes, hits or kicks them … On bad days, she seems to be here only physically. I recommend … individual attention."

Robin had adverse reactions to all the current drugs for hyperactivity. With Cylert she seemed calmer, but she couldn't sleep. She was awake twenty out of twenty-four hours. When taking Ritalin, she would shake as if freezing cold when anything moved around her—that was scary. Robin's . pediatrician considered these negative reactions and he took Robin off the drugs. We were back to the only thing we'd found to help Robin's behaviors: diet.

We did not succeed in finding an appropriate school program for Robin that year. Within one year, we had to remove her from three separate private schools. Obviously, regular mainstream placement was not the answer for her education at that time.

Five to Eleven Years Old

I remember Robin's first contact with the public school system as if it were yesterday. I requested an evaluation. There was no way Robin could go into a regular class like her sisters.

After introductions, William E. Connelly, the special education intake person, said Robin *would* go into a regular classroom. She wore a Raggedy Ann dress (which I had made), along with short white lace socks and black patent leather shoes. I was disappointed he couldn't see through her appearance. I asked how long he needed her, and I said, "I'll be back."

William E. Connelly, Prince William County Schools, Robin 5 years old

Behavioral Observations:

"She did not appear to be afraid of the examiner nor did she mind leaving her mother. Robin was extremely active throughout the testing period. She was highly distractible and it was difficult to get her to focus on a given task … Robin also demonstrated behavior suggesting that she may have a great deal of internal aggression … Robin was able to say some words but rarely used sentences. Often she would speak at the examiner rather than to him … she necessitated frequent and immediate reinforcements.

"Robin's behavior in testing suggests that while she is obviously impulsive and distractible, she also has a relatively low frustration tolerance. She seems to depend totally on external sources for whatever controls she uses and does not seem to be capable of functioning independently. She seems to have little or no idea of how to satisfy basic needs, avoid serious danger, or how to interact with others. She may also have difficulty, at times, distinguishing between herself and the world around her. Her perception of reality seems to be distorted.

"Robin seems perfectly content to remain in her own world. One gets the impression that Robin may resent the intrusion … and prefer to remain detached from others. Indeed reports of social interactions indicate that she may be trying to drive others away from her … her fine motor skills lag in development because of her high level of distractibility and impulsivity."

When I returned, Mr. Connelly agreed Robin had serious problems. I told him about all the positive changes we'd seen with her special diet and at Muriel Humphrey School. After evaluating her, he explained to me that she was emotionally *retarded*. He assured me she was not emotionally *disturbed* and that her behaviors were not the result of bad parenting. Having clarified the difference, he felt the best, and *only*, school placement they had was an Emotionally Disturbed (ED) special education class. He said he would write specific recommendations to the teacher for Robin's needs. I was just thankful for his help.

The school system required all students and their families who had a child in ED classes to be clients of the Prince William County Mental Health Department. Zeena Zeidberg, MA, was the counselor assigned for our family's home program. Ms. Zeidberg is the first person who suggested the word *autism* to us. She'd worked with children who had autism in the past.

Two days after the school year started, Mr. Connelly and Ms. Zeidberg agreed that Robin's ED public school placement was not appropriate—even with an ED teacher, aide, and only two other children in a self-contained classroom. The teacher said she couldn't handle Robin because of her behaviors and that she didn't have an attention span.

The county placed Robin that year at a private special education day school in an adjoining county. It was a one-hour bus ride from our home—each way. This placement was overwhelming for Robin, and she did not continue the progress she had made while at Muriel Humphrey School. For reinforcement, a teacher from Muriel Humphrey, Erna Gilker, tutored Robin that whole year in speech. In addition, she recommended home assignments to encourage development and language at home.

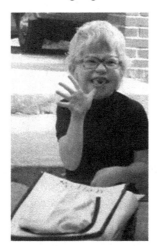

Fig. 1.3. Robin at five years old going to private school.

I wanted Robin's school placement closer to home and in the public school system. We sold our dream home in the suburbs and bought a small farm on the other end of the same county, after receiving assurances that we would find better public schools.

Robin's first public school placement in our new farming community that year was in another ED class. Mr. Connelly knew this teacher and was confident she could help Robin. I worked closely with her for support. I made sure diet-safe foods were always available; however, Robin's diet wasn't a medically approved intervention for behaviors, and therefore the school staff did not always make it a priority.

I convinced myself that, just maybe, improvements we saw in Robin resulting from this diet really were in my mind. Why was I working so hard when the school didn't seem to care? During the Christmas holidays I stopped the diet. The girls and I went wild with holiday baking; we used colored sprinkles, cake mixes, and other non-safe diet foods.

With the holidays over, the girls returned to school. Within two weeks—after an incident in the classroom with Robin eating crayons under the table—the teacher called me for help. Robin was in crisis. I told her I'd taken Robin off the diet because they were not supporting her dietary needs. They had been giving Robin non-safe treats during the day. The teacher requested I put Robin back on the diet, and she wrote this letter regarding her observations on diet intervention.

Susan Prather, Teacher ED-1, Robin 6 years old

"When Robin was on the Feingold diet, behavior management techniques worked effectively in controlling her behavior. Through the use of a variety of behavior modification techniques (token economy, verbal praise, positive touching, time out, etc.), Robin could maintain behavior conducive to instruction. Progress was made academically and behaviorally.

"Progress was halted after the Feingold diet was stopped. Robin had difficulty keeping on task even on a one-to-one relationship. Her communication skills regressed. I found her to be disoriented, tired, demanding, defensive, easily frustrated, and whiny. There was an increase in her mimicking behavior. Robin became increasingly fascinated with 'touching' things. She spent a lot of time 'feeling' the paste, water, and her own saliva. Most difficult was her lack of motivation. Previous management techniques proved futile.

"Upon placing Robin back on the Feingold diet, she slowly overcame these difficulties. Robin is progressing at the same rate previously seen before the omission of the Feingold diet..."

Robin was a very immature six year old. Her ED class consisted of emotionally disturbed ten-year-old boys, except for one other girl. Therefore, the following year, when Robin was seven, the public school system recommended a transfer to a Language Delayed/Learning Disability class. I agreed this was a better fit, but Robin's behaviors sabotaged that placement. The following year, Robin was transferred to a Learning Disability class, and the year after that back to a different Language Delayed/Learning Disabled class.

Robin had her second eye surgery during this time, but it seemed to make no difference in her academics or behaviors. All school assignments were incomplete or she received failing grades. A behavior notebook went from home to school and back daily. Robin still had more bad days than good days, and her diagnosis varied yearly. Evaluations included "emotionally retarded" as well as "mild," "moderate," or "severe retardation."

Each of these placements was in a different public school, with a different teacher and a different principal. Each school was an hour bus ride each way from our home. Robin's language therapy was fifteen minutes one or two days a week, and occupational therapy sensory integration (OT/SI) was hit-or-miss at each school.

I took my responsibility as Robin's mother very seriously, making sure she was in bed every night on time and that the child I sent to school every morning was the best she could be. To eliminate stress in the classroom, the teachers often asked me to drive Robin to school, thinking the hour-long bus ride was contributing to her behavior. I always did.

Robin's sensory deficiencies were a major issue and it was something I could focus on outside her academic settings. We filed a special education due process hearing for Robin to receive OT/SI on a regular basis through the school system. She began receiving OT/SI twice a week, after school, at the special education building. Each session was forty-five minutes, and it included a home program for reinforcement. I was more than happy to provide free transportation.

The school psychologists continually reinforced Robin's learning needs to the teachers. Some of her teachers didn't understand what Robin needed, while others didn't believe they could make a difference in her in one year. When Robin finally had a teacher who did meet her needs, the teacher didn't have the administrative authorization to develop the necessary program.

Robin was now nine years old. She'd had more than eleven evaluations, and academically she was still at the prekindergarten level. Her school time was divided between her inappropriate behaviors and simply staring into space. Many teachers felt she had *staring seizures*, because at times she seemed unaware of her surroundings or was unresponsive to stimuli.

Moving Beyond the Public School System

One of these teachers, Mrs. Hartley, along with Robin's speech therapist, opened the medical community doors for our family. They recommended that Robin have a full evaluation at Children's Hospital National Medical Center, Speech and Hearing Department, Washington, D.C.—if we could pay for it. They put us in touch with Sharon Murray, PhD. Robin had a neurological, psychological, psychiatric, and language evaluation. Her CAT scan[3] was normal but her EEG[4] showed abnormalities.

Based on Robin's EEG results, Children's Hospital medical team recommended we keep her away from strobe lights—as their rapid blinking might cause seizures. They felt she did not need medication. The psychiatrist prescribed Robin Dexedrine for behavior intervention. Within a month, she developed continual clicking sounds with her tongue and throat. The psychiatrist said this was a negative reaction and we had to take Robin off the medication.

This medical team was encouraging. Dr. Murray was impressed with Robin's obvious desire to please me during her intake evaluation. She felt this was a very good sign. Dr. Murray told us not to give up on Robin and that we could make a difference in her future. After our team meeting with all the results of these evaluations, I asked Dr. Murray why they did not label Robin as autistic. Dr. Murray looked at me as if to say, "You do not want a label." I knew she was right. A label would only limit Robin's potential and opportunities at this time in her life.

Armed with this complete team evaluation, I took Robin back to Edwin Carter, PhD, a clinical psychologist from Springfield, Virginia. He was the school psychologist when Robin attended special education private school at five years old. This time, he was able to give Robin the Wechsler Intelligence Scale for Children-Revised (WISC-R) IQ test. Robin scored 59, which indicates mental retardation. He supported Dr. Murray's evaluation for Robin's future and started us on our journey for change.

Edwin N. Carter, PhD, Clinical Psychologist, Robin 11 years old

"Because of her multitude of problems, day-to-day functioning is very difficult for Robin but she obviously is able to establish commerce [understanding] with others, the quality of it is quite poor.

---

3   Computed Axial Tomography.
4   Electroencephalogram.

"She needs a highly sheltered classroom and home environment for at least the next few years. With intensive educational experience provided by a wide variety of professionals including teachers, psychologists, speech and language therapists, and occupational therapists … I think we can look forward to some real improvement in overall functioning."

I wanted to believe Dr. Murray's team and Dr. Carter's confirmation of their prognosis for Robin. I was well aware that Robin's behaviors were best when I was her guide or instructor. She was very dependent on me for communication and she did a lot of things at home that I considered age appropriate, but not at school.

Robin started menstruating at eleven years of age. When I saw Dr. Carter at our next visit, I told him with disbelief. He stood up from his desk and said, "Great, let's get those hormones moving!" He assured me this was a positive thing for Robin's growth and development. Her periods were very regular, heavy, and confusing to her, and they lasted a full seven days!

I was still looking for that magic pill to make things easier for Robin. Her good day/bad day syndrome was heightened the week *before* her period, the week *of* her period, and the week *after* her period. That left her one week out of four that she was focused and in good spirits.

Robin and I took the shuttle to New York to see Harold Levinson, MD, author of *The Solution to the Riddle—Dyslexia* (Springer-Verlag Publisher, 1980). I read his book and I thought he could help Robin. Dr. Levinson was using Dramamine as part of his treatment plan to calm the brain. He was the first person to introduce Robin to the world of vitamins. His treatment plan for Robin used Marezine and it seemed to help her stay more consistent with clearer thinking. In addition, she was still on the Feingold diet.

I knew Robin could learn. She sat with me during the church service at our small community church. I was able to keep her busy by teaching her to compare the hymnbook numbers, listed on a board at the front of the sanctuary, and bookmark them appropriately in the hymnbook. I taught her to match page numbers from the weekly church bulletin and bookmark them appropriately in the pew books. I took prekindergarten workbooks for her to do during the sermon. Her behavior was appropriate during these exercises and she could follow my instructions.

I decided to experiment and teach Robin on Sunday mornings while Bob took Pam and Karen to Sunday school and church. This gave us over two hours a week *alone* in the house with no interruptions. I took all Robin's incomplete and failing school reproduced worksheets and retyped them as our lessons. I omitted the cutesy pictures and simplified the format, sometimes making one page into two. I needed to know whether she could really learn developmentally within a specialized environment.

Probably the most significant thing I did was to let Robin take the lead in learning. I didn't rush her, and I gave her time to complete each assignment. She had my complete attention. We sat side by side, and I encouraged positive behavior just as I'd done in church.

- Robin's printing was very poor. I helped her trace letters on the page and then she found the flash card that matched.
- Robin couldn't read so we played games with picture identification, such as Concentration.
- With math, I used real forks instead of pictures on a worksheet of forks. We added and subtracted them. She would then find the multiple choice answer.

She was amazing! This was not rote memorization or guessing. She was *learning* and really enjoyed these Sunday mornings together. I couldn't believe how easy it was to teach her. As the school year ended, we continued these learning sessions during the summer.

Since Robin couldn't learn by osmosis, her teachers said she couldn't learn. We felt the only thing limiting Robin's potential was the lack of an appropriate education. We knew her best and we were only asking for their psychologist's recommendations:

William E. Connelly, Prince William County School, Robin 11 years old

"Adaptive Behavior: Basically, Robin has mastered the self-help skills expected for an individual her age. However, there are some areas of weakness which involve socialization with her age group—this occurs primarily because of her limited communication skills and tendency to withdraw.

"Classroom Behavior: Robin functions best in settings which are highly structured, directed, and supportive. She needs firm guidance in her work, otherwise she will give up because it's difficult for her to search for an answer and find an effective way to communicate it. Robin requires considerable support and encouragement in her academic endeavors. She frustrates easily, becomes easily discouraged, and then withdraws unless she feels supported.

"Interpretation of Test Results: Robin's scores fall consistently within the Educable Mentally Retarded (EMR) range of intelligence … scores should be interpreted carefully because of her low level of tolerance for frustration … Robin has to develop a problem-solving strategy each time she is faced

with a problem to solve … Robin seems to need to learn how to apply the academic skills as well as just acquire them."

After all the positive recommendations from our private evaluations, the public school system decided to transfer Robin to our county's segregated special education building. "In this new placement," they said, "she will shine."

"No," I said, "absolutely not." We'd come too far with Robin's behaviors to accept yet another inappropriate educational placement. I wasn't giving up on Robin. She deserved a chance to learn—an education.

Twelve to Eighteen Years Old

Robin did not attend the segregated special education school building that fall, as the school system recommended. Instead, believing in Robin, we place her back at Accotink Academy, Springfield, Virginia, a special education private day school one hour from our home. Dr. Carter worked closely with the school and monitored Robin's program. She had one hour of occupational therapy sensory integration and one hour of speech-language therapy (SLT) every day before she went to her academic classroom. The changes we saw from this approach in her learning were exciting. She was having growth *spurts* in everything.

One year at Accotink was enough for our family to realize we were moving in the right direction. That year gave us time to regroup and make plans for Robin's future—which did not include the public school system.

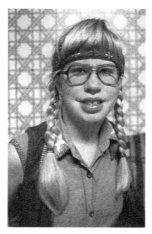

Fig. 1.4. Robin working on a home school project.

I home schooled for the next five years. Pam and Karen were away at college, and Robin and I had the house to ourselves during the day. Dr. Carter and Dr. Murray allowed me to observe Robin's evaluations to help me understand how to teach her. With their support, I realized Robin would never improve on her testing scores if she didn't have a rounded, academic education that included science, history, and geography. For example:

- What direction does the sun come up?
- What season does snow fall?
- What did Christopher Columbus do?

Robin needed to relate to other people as she did to me. She needed an academic program, but she also needed an intense coordinated program that included sensory integration, behavior, and language. This, I thought, was the true magnitude of her developmental issues. Dr. Carter had additional priorities for Robin—self-image and socialization. I started scanning our local newspaper and found two opportunities. Robin joined a local majorette corps and 4-H. On the advice of a friend, I purchased the Calvert Home School curriculum.[5]

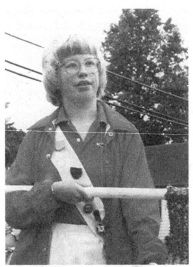

Fig. 1.5. Robin marching as a banner carrier.

For the next five years I home schooled. Robin's intense program included positive behavior modification, OT/SI, SLT, academic education, and socialization activities (see related chapters).

---

5   www.calvertschool.org.

Robin advanced in educational testing from prekindergarten to the sixth-grade level, with some testing at the tenth-grade level during this time. Her goal was to work in an office someday. I slowly withdrew her Feingold diet and the Marezine because she seemed to be doing so well. She completed Calvert third, fourth, and fifth grade curriculums. During Robin's five years of home schooling, Dr. Carter and Dr. Murray monitored her progress. She saw Dr. Carter weekly, then twice a month, while she saw Dr. Murray annually.

Edwin Carter, PhD, Clinical Psychologist, Robin 15 years old

"There are many types of skills, if learned, can result in Robin neutralizing her disorder … Robin often times feels inadequate and incompetent to deal with the demands of the world around her.

"Her low self-esteem and poor self-image plague her and often times rob her of the motivation to deal with others. She is often times too tentative in social situations unless she has the opportunity to 'rehearse' what it is that she is going to say."

Returning to Public School

Robin *wanted* to graduate from high school. She *wanted* the cap and gown experience just like her sisters. She *wanted* to go to school with her social group peers in 4-H and the majorette corps. She *needed* to get away from her mother.

Robin went to our local public high school—five minutes away from our house—for her last two years in school. She loved the routine. She managed the confusion of lunch and changing classes without incident. Robin's learning disability (LD) teacher gave her one-on-one instruction for the Virginia Tenth Grade State Competency Test. Robin passed both tests— reading and math. Robin's teachers were very supportive of her program and they made a genuine effort to include Robin in school and classroom activities.

Robin walked down the aisle with her majorette and 4-H peers and graduated from high school with a Certificate of Attendance. She was eighteen years old.

Adulthood: Nineteen Years Old to the Present

After graduating from high school, Robin became a volunteer for the National Vaccine Information Center (NVIC), a non-profit organization. I was the executive director and had set up their office in Pam and Karen's old bedrooms while Robin was in high school. In one bedroom I had networked computers, and the other was the mail and copy center.

Robin's autism was definitely an asset in the office environment. We had separate responsibilities, yet she stayed focused, consistent, organized, and accurate at all times with me as her guide. She opened and read all the mail, paper-clipped each letter's contents, and stacked them organized by each check's dollar amount. We had a lot of mail, and she enjoyed briefing me on their contents. I answered the mail, put the information into the computer database, and coded the checks for Robin to enter into Quicken, and she wrote the deposit slips. I took her to the bank so she could deposit the checks. She would get very upset if anyone tried to open the mail or look for vaccine articles in the *Journal of the American Medical Association* (JAMA). That was *her* job.

Robin attended many Health and Human Service (HHS) and Institute of Medicine (IOM) vaccine-related meetings with me. She knew all the professionals in these meetings and they knew her. It was a very busy time working with families, doctors, attorneys, press, and legislators. We hired another person to work in the office, and we kept this schedule until our planned move to Florida, when Robin was twenty-two years old.

Moving to Florida

Robin was excited about our move (1993). My main requirement in our house-hunting was sidewalks. We found a house with sidewalks on the same side of the street as a shopping center under construction. *Maybe she can walk to the store someday,* I thought. We joined the local church and enjoyed going to the beach.

Robin was having a lot of trouble adjusting to our retirement life. She wasn't used to Bob being home all the time. Bob focused on Robin accepting him as part of our life changes. In order to stay positive, they started taking tai chi classes together.

As months passed, we found ourselves tiptoeing around Robin's behaviors—anger, anxiousness, and frustration. She seemed depressed and bored. She was losing basic language skills and once again withdrawing back into her *own world*. When overwhelmed, she headed to her bedroom, often slamming the door. She was exhausting. Pam and Karen's lives were moving forward while Robin was moving backwards. I was fearful that her baby doctors were right—she was regressing.

Robin felt important in her volunteer office job at NVIC when we lived in Virginia, and I thought that perhaps she needed a real job. I did some research and requested a state employment evaluation. Robin received a six-week evaluation through our local Association for Retarded Citizens (ARC). However, they did not encourage employment for her at this time.

We were determined not to give up and she finally got her first job bagging groceries in a local supermarket (see chapter 8: Employment).

Robin started Tae Kwon Do classes at our local YMCA. She was in a class with ten-year-old boys. This certainly wasn't age appropriate, but she loved it, and the teacher was great with her. YMCA staff cheered her on for success—eventually she got her red belt. Years later she enrolled in age appropriate karate. She has a blue belt in karate.

Another mother and I started a social group for young adults, Mainstreamed Adult Singles at Home (MASH). MASH targeted challenged adults living at home who wanted to be a part of their community. Many of these young adults already had jobs; they just needed a social connection (see chapter 6: Socialization and Self-Image).

I learned from my fellow MASH mothers that Florida offered state services (companion, therapies, and group homes) for individuals with developmental disabilities. I was very interested, because I felt Robin desperately needed additional language therapy.

We felt Robin should qualify for state services in Florida. It was her only hope for a future. Even without a label, we knew she was a case of classic autism. We returned to Virginia and Dr. Carter gave us the necessary evaluation of "autistic." We were now sure that we were within the law, but the state did not accept her admission. Robin was denied services.

Edwin N. Carter, PhD, Clinical Psychologist, Robin 28 years old

"I have known Robin for over twenty years and recently had the opportunity to re-evaluate her in my Virginia office. It is my opinion that Robin should be diagnosed as an autistic child. She has shown the symptoms associated with this diagnosis since I first evaluated her in the late 1970s, manifesting, for example, communication problems when she appears to have enough intelligence to be able to communicate at a higher level. Further, she demonstrates the socially inappropriate, isolated thinking, and limited skills of autonomy associated with autism…"

Unable to understand why we were having problems, I called the Center for Autism and Related Disabilities (CARD) in Florida for help. They gave me a list of psychiatrists and I made an appointment for Robin. After evaluating Robin, Dr. Morales requested Robin's past psychological evaluations—all twenty. She agreed that Robin qualified as *classic autism*:

Alice Morales, MD, PA, Psychiatric Evaluation, Robin 28 years old

"I have reviewed Ms. Millan's [extensive] prior evaluations, and after reading these … it is evident that as a child she met the criteria for autism but was never given that diagnosis. It is also clear that her IQ increased each year due to rote memorization of the text. However, she functions on a mentally retarded level and without her parents' continued and constant support, she would function on a much lower level.

Axis I: Autistic
Axis II: Mild mental retardation with developmental reading disorder
Axis III: Two eye surgeries to correct strabismus
Axis IV: Severe/chronic psychiatric problems, severe anxiety disorder
Axis V: GAF—50"

Robin began receiving services through the Florida Home and Community Based Services (HCBS) Medicaid waiver when she was twenty-eight years old.[6] She began language therapy three hours a week.

With all this in place for Robin, she was still having problems with mental drifting and erratic behaviors. I was afraid she was going to lose her job at Publix bagging groceries. We couldn't seem to stabilize her thinking, behavior, and motivation all at the same time. I was still dealing with my biggest fear—regression.

I decided to put Robin back on the Marezine she'd taken when I home schooled. We did see some positive results. She seemed to think more clearly and she had more energy.

Continuing my search for Robin's stabilization in her adulthood, Bob, Robin, and I attended a one-day conference on the biomedical treatments of autism. I wanted to personally meet with and hear the speakers talk about their autism research. Leaving this conference, Bob and I knew this is what we needed to do to help Robin (see chapter 2: Diet, Vitamins, and Supplements).

Following the conference, we made an appointment with Jeff Bradstreet, MD. He requested we put Robin on the gluten-free casein-free diet before her appointment. At her appointment he started Robin on the hormone

---

6   Federal and state partnership with the Centers for Medicaid and Medicare Services (CMS).

secretin, along with vitamins and supplements. He supported Robin's need for additional language therapy and encouraged her development as an adult.

This time, Robin's growth *spurts* were moving faster than Bob and I could keep up. Her smile and her positive attitude both returned. She was no longer angry all the time and arguing with us about everything. Her energy level returned and we began seeking out additional social activities. Transportation is a serious issue where we lived and Robin was dependent on us for her transportation.

We went through the Department of Vocational Rehabilitation (VR) to find a professional instructor to help Robin get her driver's license. The instructor was very patient with her. After his driving lessons (and a lot of reinforcement from us), she eventually got her license. That was the easy part. It took another year before she drove anywhere by herself, except to work.

Originally, I was concerned about the road rage of other drivers. My concerns were misplaced, as it was Robin who had the road rage. She would get mad if a traffic light turned red when she was going through it, or when somebody went over the speed limit, or when someone followed her too closely. We were patient when it came to helping her understand responsible driving, riding as her passengers almost everywhere she went.

The cashier supervisor at Publix asked Robin if she wanted to be a cashier now that she had her driver's license. Of course, Robin's answer was yes. Robin had one big problem, however: she didn't understand money. Motivation is a very powerful thing, and she soon learned this as well.

With encouragement from Robin's HCBS waiver coordinator, Bob and I had a serious talk with Robin about independent living. We felt she deserved this chance. Robin wanted her own home, like her sisters. Her coordinator helped us find a housing loan and a state-supported living coach. The coach's purpose was to help Robin with her scheduling, cleaning, and daily life activities (see chapter 10: Moving Out: Independent Living).

Robin moved into her own condominium one week before her thirtieth birthday—two miles from our house. She had to give up her piano lessons and the martial arts, as she could no longer afford those costly luxuries. Robin's cousin gave her a kitten, Snowball, for a roommate.

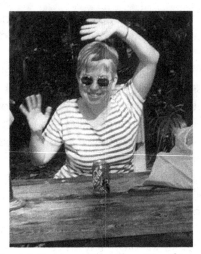

Fig. 1.6. Robin acting silly with a friend.

Fortunately for Robin, she wants us in her life. Independent living wasn't easy for her at first, and there were many challenges for everyone. I'm still Robin's best communicator, but that is rapidly changing. Her current language therapist has been able to help her comfortably express herself more appropriately (see chapter 4: Speech and Language Therapy).

Robin will always have autism, including social, intellectual, and language disabilities, but these do not limit her options as an adult. At thirty-eight years old, she doesn't see any of this as a disability, and neither do the people around her. Her autism is stabilized with biomedical interventions, Marezine, and language therapy.

Robin's a lot of fun and she's definitely her own person. She's been in her condominium for eight years now and employed at Publix for fifteen years. Three years ago she started a second job as membership receptionist at our local YMCA. Although she's a part of the community around her, her closest friends are in her social group, MASH. She and Jonathan have been dating for over a year.

PART II
Embracing the Many Modes of Treatment

I don't need your pity, I need your help!

—Ann Millan

Chapter 2:
Diet, Vitamins, and Supplements

The Relationship between Food and Mood

Robin's immune system seemed excellent. She had no apparent allergies. She was never sick, and her weight gain was normal. Her digestive and bowel systems seemed fine. Robin was our healthiest child. Her sister Pam had environmental allergies (grass, mold, trees) and both Pam and Karen spent their younger years fighting ear infections and tonsillitis. I've also had environmental allergies and chronic eczema since childhood.

When Robin was a baby, we'd do anything to stop her screaming. At four years old, it was still our major focus, along with her constant running. We'd tried all the behavior management prescription drugs without success. She had side effects to all of them.

Given the general good state of her health, Robin's up-and-down behaviors (good day/bad day syndrome) made no sense to us. She was exhausting. She would dig her hand harder and harder into her mouth, as she bit down on it while running.

Trying to help us, a neighbor brought me a *People* magazine, dated December 8, 1975. It contained an article about the Feingold diet, which said that it was possible to change a child's behavior by eliminating food colorings and preservatives in the diet.

Was Robin affected by the food she ate? Could food have been causing her good-day/bad-day syndrome?

I made an appointment with Robin's pediatrician. He strongly disapproved of diet intervention and he would not support me. He said it was voodoo medicine. Obviously, he didn't see my desperate need for help! Following my instincts, I read *Why Your Child Is Hyperactive* by Benjamin Feingold, MD (Random House, 1975) and started Robin on the diet. She was four years old.

Within a week on the diet, Robin stopped biting her hand while running and her screaming went down an octave. We couldn't believe it! We finally found something that helped. It didn't solve all her problems, but it helped. Baby steps were survival for us.

As months went by, her senses (sight, sound, touch) began to develop. We finally felt we had a child who might be able to communicate. She was beginning to listen. She stopped kicking her sisters. She slept through the night without rocking or outbursts of screaming. She sat at the kitchen table for the first time. She traveled well in the car and we could take her shopping. For simplicity's sake, the whole family ate Robin's Feingold-safe food. We never ate non-diet food in front of her—ever!

I was determined to succeed. I kept the recommended diet diary, comparing food to mood. I became a detective, writing everything down and comparing previous notes when Robin had a good or bad day. I even compared mornings to afternoons to evenings. When Robin did have flare-ups in her behavior, I used my diary to isolate foods I thought might be the triggers and started over again. If I hadn't kept this diary, I don't think I would have noticed the subtle changes in her development.

When I realized I could control Robin's behavior, I became compulsive about her diet. I was so excited. My focus was on what Robin could eat, not only what she couldn't eat. Reading labels and substituting food brands was difficult. Food labels had foreign initials and words I was not familiar with. Some labels, on foods like macaroni, cocoa, and butter, didn't even list ingredients.

Robin was on the Feingold diet for twelve years (from four to sixteen). She blossomed at home but not in public school. Our home life became her haven as she was fitting into our family activities. She enjoyed the farm animals and all the outside activities when we moved to the farm. She had a lot of energy and we kept her busy and focused on the things around her.

As I was finalizing Robin's home schooling when she was fifteen, I slowly added non-safe Feingold foods back into her diet. She seemed stabilized through behavior modification, Marezine, vitamins, and her home school program. I felt I needed to stop treating her as *special* around her peers, because she was going back to public school. Her self-image was my priority. In her social activities, she needed to eat at parties and order meals from a restaurant's menu, like other people did.

Although I continued using many Feingold-safe foods in my kitchen, Robin had no dietary restrictions for the next twelve years. Admittedly, I was seeing flexible behavior in her daily life, but I had long ago forgotten about her good-day/bad-day syndrome or diet intervention.

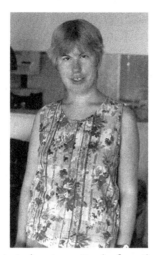

Fig. 2.1. Robin in her twenties before the GFCF diet.

At twenty-eight years old, Robin hadn't been bouncing back from her regressive episodes for some time. I feared she was in a state of perpetual regression. She had consistent problems with mental drifting and erratic behavior—anxiety, anger, and frustration. When frustrated with us, she would stomp into her bedroom and slam the door. I was concerned this might happen at work and she'd lose her job.

Bob, Robin, and I attended a one-day conference on the biomedical treatments of autism—the gluten-free casein-free (GFCF) diet along with vitamins and supplements. I'd been reading the Autism Research Institute (ARI) newsletter for many years and watching the Defeat Autism Now (DAN) protocol emerging. I was curious and wanted to personally meet and hear the speakers talk about their research. Andrew Wakefield, MD, a gastroenterologist from the Royal Free Hospital Medical School in London, spoke about toxicity of metals and chemical sensitivity in children. He had found that some children's guts (stomach) were leaking poisons into their brain and this poison may be causing many of the autism behaviors in some children. The focus, he said, should be on healing the gut and balancing the immune system. Other speakers said children with autism have a poor immune system and could not process nutrients properly.

The conference was very motivational and exciting. Parents and doctors filled the audience, listening to success after success of children with autism on this biomedical intervention. However, they were only talking about children, whereas Robin was now twenty-eight years old.

I knew it was going to be difficult getting Robin's cooperation to go back on a diet. I turned to her during the session and said, "Do you want to go back on a diet and try to get your driver's license?" I was always goal oriented, and it was the most motivational thing I could think of. We discussed it and she said yes. I made an appointment with Jeff Bradstreet, MD, International Child Development Resource Center (ICDRC), Melbourne, Florida.

Dr. Bradstreet asked me to put Robin on the GFCF diet before our initial appointment, and I did.

After two weeks on this new diet, with no additional vitamins or supplements, Pam's family came for a visit. We took all the buckets and shovels and headed for Clearwater Beach. Robin had perfected the art of appearing socially acceptable yet not relating to others. Yet on this day, Pam and I suddenly realized Robin was in the middle of her kids playing. This was the very first time Robin had independently played with anyone without continual prompting. I took pictures of this event and a framed, enlarged copy hangs on our bedroom wall.

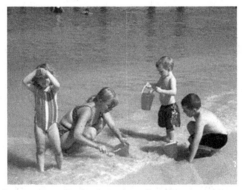

Fig. 2.2. The first time Robin played with anyone without prompting.

When we saw Dr. Bradstreet, I excitedly showed him the picture. He was pleased that we'd seen changes in Robin with the diet. After his evaluation, he started her off with the hormone secretin, along with fish oil, folic acid, B-6, and B-12 vitamins. Later, he added glutathione, which resulted in another giant leap in Robin's development. From there he added another set of supplements for cell repair.

Within two years on DAN, Robin had that driver's license and much more. She had her guardianship rights restored, got a promotion to cashier at Publix supermarket, and moved into her own condominium. Robin has been Dr. Bradstreet's patient for over ten years. He sees her annually. She's on the GFCF diet 80 percent of the time now and seems to be doing fine with this change. She faithfully takes her supplements daily.

The Feingold Diet

The Feingold diet focuses on removing artificial colors, flavors, and preservatives from the diets of hyperactive children. If parents do not see positive results in their child, Dr. Feingold also recommends removing salicylates from their diet. (Salicylates, present in many fruits, create a chemical similar to aspirin.) I also eliminated salicylates, hoping for faster progress.

With the Feingold diet, I had to cook most things from scratch. I focused on volume cooking and freezing. I'd fry forty chicken legs and freeze them for Robin's lunches or snacks. I think the most desperate thing I ever did was to make my own mayonnaise. My biggest problem was liquids, because Robin was a heavy drinker. Several times I switched to goat's milk, thinking the process of pasteurization might be causing reactions. Our neighbor gave us goat's milk every morning and another neighbor sold us butter. It was easy to go natural living in a farming community.

I didn't use expensive prepared boxed foods, so the diet didn't seem expensive to me. I did, however, have to use specific brands, not sale items, which hurt sometimes. I bought Cheerios instead of colored Fruit Loops. I bought bananas and watermelon instead of oranges and apples. My monthly *Feingold Newsletter* provided new recipes and food items available at the local grocery and health food stores.

When I helped other families start the Feingold diet, I always suggested focusing on minimum food choices the first two weeks to avoid beginner mistakes. Families need results as soon as possible to believe in diet intervention. I suggested they start by preparing their child's favorite foods, as most dishes can be adapted to fit the diet. Families using this diet will automatically return to simple, basic cooking, and many have found it easier to use organic products. Most health food stores clearly label their products, and organic foods are naturally free of MSG, nitrates, preservatives, artificial flavorings and colorings, and a host of unpronounceable chemicals.

In addition to Dr. Feingold's book, Jane Hershey, associate director of the Feingold Association of the United States (FAUS), has written additional books to help families.[7]

GFCF Diet

The gluten-free casein-free diet, as the name suggests, eliminates the intake of glutens (naturally occurring proteins found in wheat, barley,

---

7   www.feingold.org.

spelt, triticale, kamut, rye, and possibly oats) and casein (found in all milk products).[8]

For our family, the Feingold diet was much easier to follow than the GFCF diet, because food could easily be substituted. Searching the grocery store shelves, gluten or casein was in everything. But like before, I started this diet with a determined attitude. I went back to my diet diary and kept track of food versus behaviors. I read books, labels, and more books. I went to the health store and saw that everything GFCF was at least a third more expensive than regular items. This diet did require a budget adjustment, but it was a small price to pay for our sanity.

The good news was that Robin was enjoyable again after starting the GFCF diet. She started giving us eye contact again and was more predictable and not angry all the time. Her concentration improved and she listened rather than stomping off in frustration. The bad news was that I bought a bread machine and all the different flours only to fail time and time again with the recipes. I wasted a lot of money and time by making everything too complicated.

I met a woman with celiac disease who gets very ill when she eats gluten. She invited me to a celiac support group meeting at our local hospital.[9] People with celiac disease eliminate gluten from their diet, but not milk. I could adjust to GFCF with them because I had already identified acceptable non-dairy products, for example, soy and rice milk. I went to the meeting and they helped me feel comfortable working with the diet.

That was ten years ago. Our daughter Karen and her son are now on the GFCF diet and she is my support system.

Karen's Thoughts on Diet

Today there are plenty of good GFCF baking mixes. Some are even comparably priced with traditional mixes. They are easier for a busy mother, with no surprise mistakes. However, you will become a fast learner, because product *quality* and *taste* vary greatly from brand to brand. Crepes are the only GFCF product I actually make from scratch anymore.

Food manufacturers are listening to people who are gluten intolerant. Betty Crocker now has cake and cookie mixes in most grocery stores alongside their other mixes. Sam's Club is carrying Simply Organic banana bread and carrot cake mixes. Chex corn and rice cereals and Hormel Dinty Moore Beef

---

8   www.autism.com.
9   www.celiac.org.

Stew are advertised as gluten free. Most of these items are appropriately priced, but beware—we need to make sure they are also casein free!

For breakfast, I like to start my son out with protein; however, there are many GFCF cereals, breakfast bars, and pancake mixes. I then use soy or rice milk.

For lunch, we often serve meatballs with barbeque or ketchup dipping sauce. Tuna and corn chips are also good. Sandwiches are hard. I find if I fry the bread in margarine, as if I'm making a grilled sandwich, then make the sandwich, it isn't as dry.

Dinner is basically meat and vegetables. Salads are big, of course, and I try to get creative with them. Think Mexican with corn tortillas or Asian/Indian with rice. Glutino and Amy both have gluten-free pizza with soy cheese. I often make my own pizza using the Food for Life gluten-free tortillas. I use "Follow Your Heart" Vegan Gourmet cheese. It melts.

For snacks, I make a "snack basket" for school or outings. When my son's friends have a snack, the teacher pulls out his basket from which she can choose, including individual juice packs containing 100 percent real juice. There will be pretzels, corn chips, applesauce, cereal, and a coral bar (the latter two are from EnviroKids).

GFCF foods are everywhere, including grocery stores, health food stores, and Web stores. Some products must be purchased by the case. This is where networking with others comes in handy. These are my favorite things:

- *Breads*: My two favorite breads right now are from Kinikinik and Whole Foods Market.
- *Cake mixes*: Pamela mixes are good. Their Baking and Pancake Mix is similar to Bisquick and has many uses, including pancakes, banana nut bread, and muffins. I also like all their cake and brownie mixes.
- *Cookies and snacks*: Kinikinik's KinniTOOS are the best in my book. They now have doughnuts! Their waffles are the best I've found.
- *Breakfast bars*: Mrs. May's Naturals has a chewy breakfast bar with dried fruits. Glutino also has good breakfast bars.
- *Pasta*: Tinkyada Pasta Joy. Best, in my opinion, hands down. Be sure to cook it all the way through.
- *Crackers*: Glutino, EnerG, and Mary's Gone Crackers. I like how EnerG crackers are packaged. The onion-flavored crackers are best because they don't crack and crumble like the plain ones do.

- *Eating out*: There are a number of restaurants that cater to GFCF patrons. P.F. Chang's China Bistro has a gluten-free menu, as does Outback Steakhouse. Usually we just go to organic or Asian restaurants (Thai or Vietnamese). You can buy rice or rice noodle dishes, but make sure they are GFCF. Bring your own soy sauce that doesn't contain wheat.

Obviously, I am not a medical professional. These are my thoughts and personal interpretations from my research and experiences. Always double check products—they need to say "gluten-free," and they will usually say "dairy-free" instead of casein-free. Products change, so always double check. The same thing applies to restaurants—you need both gluten-free and casein/dairy-free.

Don't give up on diet intervention too soon because the Feingold or GFCF diet does not seem to help your child. Diet counselors are very knowledgeable today and can help narrow the triggers—soy, corn, yeast, rice, or eggs— to name a few. Just look at how peanut allergies have surfaced in the last twenty years!

The question you should ask yourself when you are thinking about starting diet interventions for your child is: *Are you also sensitive?* The apple really doesn't fall far from the tree—it's just more bruised. You need to be strong and mentally clear for the battle you are about to wage for the sake of your child with autism. My mom is a good example. In just the last couple of years, to support Robin, she also started the GFCF diet even though tests results showed she was not allergic to gluten. To her amazement, her eczema cleared up. She could have saved years of pain and suffering had she just known.

We live in a world with added hormones and genetically modified products in almost everything. Consider that both potatoes and rice are highly genetically modified. Organic products will not be genetically modified. Also, hormone-free should be clearly marked on affected products.

Make your own path. Read labels. Eat simply and, if you can, locally. I always think: How did God intend for this to be eaten? We have somehow created chemical sensitivity in our population. Let's start rebuilding our health and our DNA so our children's children will be able to produce stronger, healthier children. The shortcut is rarely the best way.

Chapter 3:
Occupational Therapy
Sensory Integration (OT/SI)

Robin didn't put her hands in front of her to break a fall as she hit the ground—ever. She felt no pain, so falling really didn't matter to her. We were continually screaming, "Don't run!" trying to protect her chin as she fell. She had several rounds of stitches in the same spot from falling, and her doctors warned us she had no more skin to stitch.

Most of us never think about the automatic steps our brain takes to process information every second. The simple act of using a pencil—we just do it. For Robin, it was impossible for her to sit still in a chair, pick up a pencil, write on a piece of paper, and continue holding that pencil. She'd rather run!

Our bodies take information into our brain from many different sources in the blink of an eye. Sight, sound, smell, taste, temperature, pain, position, movement, and even the pull of gravity must all be interpreted with precision in order to generate the necessary automatic response. Educational learning, behavior, and speech will all be affected in children who have difficulty accomplishing these basic responses. The consequences can be anxiousness, frustration, anger, and confusion—words all autism parents are familiar with.

OT/SI specializes in coordinating and developing appropriate sequential sensory processing in the brain. If done properly, the brain can teach itself to develop these automatic functions. An experienced therapist is critical, because each child has different needs. Occupational therapist A. Jean Ayres, PhD, in her book *Sensory Integration and the Child* (Western Psychological Services, 1979-2005) describes SI dysfunction as a traffic jam in the brain. Some bits of sensory information get tied up in "traffic," and certain parts of the brain do not get the sensory information they need to do their jobs.

Take Nothing for Granted

Sensory integration begins before birth. The brain begins learning and forming reactions to movement in the womb. Pregnant mothers feel the rolling and twisting activity of their baby, and the baby hears their mother's voice or loud noises. Although I didn't have as much movement with Robin during pregnancy as I did with the other girls, Robin did have these responses, and my gynecologist said he was not concerned.

As an infant, Robin demanded my attention when she was awake for reasons I really didn't understand; thus we danced around the house as I held her firmly in a prone face-down position on my forearm. She seemed to be in pain, always screaming and never happy. When she was two years old, we were assigned an infant stimulation coach who encouraged us to keep her motivated and busy. When Robin was seven years old, a special education teacher suggested I investigate OT/SI. I read Dr. Ayres's book about the importance of sensory input and with this education, sensory integration became an equal partner in Robin's development for me, along with her diet and language therapy.

Robin's Sensory Deficits

Many school professionals tried to discourage me from researching OT/SI, saying Robin was too old. I finally found an OT/SI therapist who evaluated Robin and began treating her sensory issues, also giving me a home treatment plan. In Robin's SI testing, she had four critical areas of dysfunctioning deficits: attention and regulation, sensory defensiveness, behavior, and activity level.

Attention and Regulation

Attention and regulation is defined as the ability to filter through and prioritize all background noises and visual stimulation, such as determining a parent's voice over the sound of a radio or television. This is also referred to at times as "figure ground" problems.

As an example, Robin was in Mrs. Hartley's learning disability special education class when she was seven years old. Mrs. Hartley said she couldn't teach Robin with the clock hanging on the wall—it ticked and the hands moved! This was too much distraction for Robin. In addition, Robin couldn't focus on her lessons with all the distractions of the other students around her. We carpeted her classroom, hoping it would help, but there was no change.

Sensory Defensiveness

Sensory defensiveness is characterized by a fight-flight-or-fright reaction to sensory information most of us find harmless. Tactile defensiveness or hyper-responsiveness to touch is a phrase coined by Dr. Ayres. As the name implies, all senses can be involved, including tactile, auditory, visual, and vestibular (intolerance to movement).

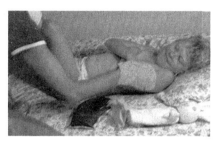

Fig. 3.1. Robin accepting touch through tactile stimulation.

Tactile: Robin screamed and ran away from us if we touched her. My first home program was to address Robin's tactile system. I made mittens of different textured materials (rough, smooth, soft, and hard) and rubbed her skin as prescribed by the therapist. The direction of rubbing was important. Robin would do the same to me. She learned to like this touching time together.

Auditory: Robin did not hear one sound, just a crowd of sounds. To get her attention, I isolated my voice while still competing with the sounds around her. I did this by firmly grasping her arm as I spoke in a normal but firm voice, using one- to two-word sentences. When I finished talking, I let go of her arm. Growing up, addressing Robin's auditory system has always been a major focus because of her many weaknesses in this area. Robin couldn't handle the sound of fireworks or a fire truck passing—it was all overwhelming for her. Only in the last couple of years has she finally been able to tell the difference between the ringing sound and the busy signal when making a telephone call.

Visual: Robin did not look at anything around her, including me. She seemed to look past us or see through us. I would try to get her to look at my face, a toy, or a blanket, but she did not see objects. My infant stimulation coach helped me realize the importance of using calming colors and putting only a few items in her bedroom at a time. When Robin was an infant, I would lay her on the floor in front of me. Then, I would slowly pull her up to my face so that I was the only thing she could see. Later, when home schooling,

I took pictures off the wall, keeping the room basic and simple. I did not use workbooks with busy pictures or too much on a page.

Vestibular: To an inexperienced person, Robin's vestibular issues might have looked like fear, in other words, psychological. Actually, they were developmental—a physical response to movements, actions, or activities moving around her that she could not process. As a baby, Robin could not tolerate being held in a normal position. As a child, she was very careful to avoid heights, including stairs, tall buildings, elevators, escalators, and balconies. She would crawl up stairs if we didn't firmly hold both hands and insist she go up. On the other hand, she loved roller coasters. These behaviors limited Robin's opportunities to appropriately socialize with her peers. As an adult, when she moved into her condominium, she was forced to address this issue because she lived on the second floor. In just the last few years, she has been able to stand at a railing and look over a balcony.

Behavior

Sensory integration dysfunction is seen in behavior patterns when a child cannot self-regulate or sequence physical tasks. The immature brain stem cannot recall responses or learn from past experience. Thus, everything seems to repeat itself, with the same consequences every time. This child will not have normal responses, including safety reflexes (e.g., putting their hands out to cushion a fall). They will not recognize the calming influence of their mother's voice or the safety of their mother's touch. As the child ages, these problems magnify into emotional and social confusion and delays.

As a child, Robin lay prone on a large ball, and the first goal was for her to automatically lift her head up to look in front of her for safety. Second, she learned to be reflexive and stop her fall, or the ball, by putting her hands out to stop. As an adult, Robin has learned to self-regulate by applying positive traits, namely compulsiveness and accuracy. For example, she once left a meeting to get something from the car and forgot to take her cell phone with her. She got lost and didn't have her phone to call for help. Finally returning to the meeting, she was angry and frustrated because I didn't come to find her. Today, Robin never forgets her cell phone. This is her way of self-regulating.

Activity Level

Activity level is often seen as developmental play. Six areas were outlined in testing, and Robin fit into each one.

1. *The child is disorganized and lacks purpose in activity.* When Robin was little, we didn't take many pictures. They reminded us of what she couldn't do. Her therapist told us it was important for Robin to understand the world around her—by using pictures. I immediately started taking pictures and organizing and sequencing them appropriately in photograph albums. I was surprised how much she enjoyed looking at herself. Even today, if we are talking about something or someone from years past, Robin will go through these old albums and find a picture of it.

2. *The child does not move around and explore the environment.* Robin hated riding in the car or anything moving around her. Trying to keep her occupied while driving, Bob always played a game with her to keep her mentally engaged. They started out identifying cars and trucks, progressing to oncoming eighteen-wheeler trucks. (Is it a Peterbilt or a Kenworth?) Her accuracy was 100 percent, and she looked forward to this game throughout the years. Personally, I never saw the difference, and I gladly sat in the back seat. As years went by, Bob had access to several large motor homes used as business labs for his job. Robin added this repertoire to her road identification talents. Today, GMC motor homes are classics, and they still spot them on the road when traveling.

3. *The child lacks variety in play activities.* Robin did not explore and she did not exhibit curiosity, an essential element to play and a brain function that elicits pleasure. Without success, I'd open the kitchen cabinet doors trying to get her to pull the pots and pans out to play with them. I remember her Barbie doll with her house, clothes, and car. Robin just sat while I played. We had to teach Robin how to be curious and pair it with something that made it desirable to repeat. Robin got this intensity from her sisters growing up. When she joined the majorette corps and 4-H, she received immediate reinforcement, with individual ribbons, certificates, or trophies following the activity.

4. *The child appears clumsy, trips easily, and has poor balance.* Robin never walked, except for support from furniture or a chair, when learning to walk. It was easier for her to run, because running didn't require balance or postural control. Robin would easily fall, and this was a problem. She was clumsy—she tripped over things on the floor or even outside. I was finally able to control Robin's running when she started the Feingold diet. To work

on her balance, I focused on coordinated body exercises in our home program—rolling, walking on planks, and coordinated crawling. I brought our hammock in the house one winter. Getting out of the hammock really seemed to raise Robin's frustration level. For more variety, I wrapped her arms and legs in toilet paper and then asked her to get out of the hammock. I was good at changing and challenging her frustrations.

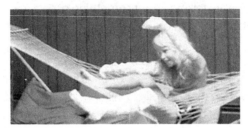

Fig. 3.2. Working on balance.

5. *The child has difficulty calming himself or herself.* Robin had no mechanism of self-comfort unless she was sleeping. She was so defensive about us touching her. As a toddler, biting her hand while running must have had a calming effect, because she always did it. She did rock and bang her head, but she didn't hold the rhythm for extended periods.

6. *The child seeks excessive amounts of vigorous sensory input.* Robin was always so rough with other people, including me. During any quiet moments together, she always ended up tickling me until I pushed her away and said, "Stop it, that hurts." Another example: Bob rushed home from a playground with blood all over Robin's face. She'd been running around from the sliding board, to the ladder, up, down, and back around repeatedly, faster and faster, until she finally fell. She was having fun, and Bob didn't realize the importance of stopping the activity before she got hurt.

OT/SI Home Program

To meet these above activity goals, and to get Robin's cooperation, I made her OT/SI home program into a *circus,* and I was the *circus master,* encouraging her participation. We pushed the furniture against the walls to create a path in our family room. Robin would lie on the floor, arms straight above her head, and roll from one end of the room to the other. She kept veering off the path, because her body strength was not equal on both sides. The goal was to stay straight on the path. This was very difficult for her.

Both sides of Robin's brain were not working together. Robin would pick up a glass of milk with her left hand if the glass was on the left side of her plate at the table. If the glass was on the right side of the plate, she would pick it up with her right hand. The brain crossing over from side to side or at midline is a very important part of brain development. Both sides of Robin's brain were not communicating. They were functioning separately from each other—not a good thing.

An exercise to encourage her brain to cross at midline was the use of a scooter board. Robin would sit on the board, cross her legs in front of her (Indian style), and put her hands on the floor to turn the board in circles. At first, both hands pushed *parallel* together to make the circle. Eventually, trying to spin faster, she automatically *crossed* one hand over the other. We did this to the left and then to the right. Both sides of Robin's brain were now working as a team, crossing midline.

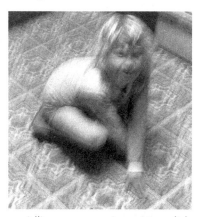

Fig. 3.3. Crossing midline was a major accomplishment for Robin.

Another performance in our circus was to play *wheelbarrow*. The goal was for me to hold Robin's feet up in the air as she walked on her hands down the circus runway. Robin didn't have the strength to do this, so she dragged her body as she balanced her weight on her elbows and forearms. She raced in this position from one end of the family room to the other. Because this was a race, she eventually pulled herself up to move faster. She still had the left hand on the left side, right hand on the right side. As months passed and we tried to beat her previous speed, she automatically began to cross her left hand over to the right side and then her right hand over to the left side. Success!

Walking with a book on her head, standing on one foot, and counting how long she could hold it became a game. This activity had a lot of progressive variety. We could hop in the same spot, hop moving forward, or hop in circles. This was fun for her, because I couldn't do it either.

OT/SI Home School Program

I continued Robin's daily OT/SI private school program when I began home schooling. It was designed by their therapist, who finally felt comfortable allowing me to incorporate spinning into my program. I followed her instructions, because I knew spinning could be very dangerous if not monitored and done properly.

I started every morning with OT/SI. Bob put a swivel hook in the middle of the family room ceiling for an OT swing. This swing was a piece of plywood, covered with carpet and suspended from the ceiling by ropes. Robin would lay flat, face-down on her stomach or face-up on her back. It was important her spinal cord was straight. I followed our new OT's recommendations by slowly spinning right, then left, then slowly swinging back and forth. Even though Robin was afraid of heights, she liked the swing.

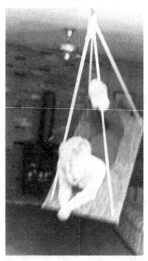

Fig. 3.4. Robin on her therapy swing.

While spinning, we talked about the day's schedule, reviewed multiplication tables, and did other homework. It was very calming for her, and it made a difference in her day. She could definitely focus better after these sessions.

Robin skipped. Skipping with consistency was very difficult. She loved to skip from one end of the house to the other. After skipping, we had a scavenger hunt. I placed masking tape arrows all through the house, up, over, and under furniture. I mixed up the task daily. She liked the scavenger hunts.

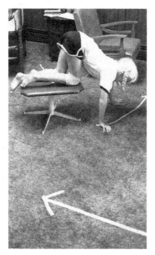

Fig. 3.5. A treasure hunt to incorporate gross motor skills.

Settling down for lessons, we started by playing *Simon*. This was a popular game in the 1980s and still is today. When Robin pushed the start button, it initiated a lighted color with sound, and she had to duplicate the color/sound/rhythm combination. The game built on that color/sound/rhythm combo to include another step, and another. We would do it together, and I would point to the correct button if she had trouble. When we won a game, lights and sounds went haywire. Eventually we went from sharing the same game to competing against each other.

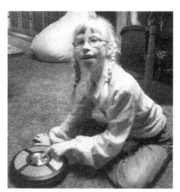

Fig. 3.6. Robin learning to sequence.

Variety was important. Robin liked the gross (big) motor skill activities. I had read they were important before working on the fine (small) motor skills, like writing. I found Glass Wax, a product for cleaning windows, years ago. I'd let the film dry on our sliding glass door, and Robin would write and draw in the film. Whenever she had problems with school lessons, like writing a specific letter, we practiced writing it on the door. Robin loved waking up in the mornings and writing in the dew on the windows—she also learned how to clean windows.

The more we did, the more I thought of. I needed lots of things to keep Robin busy, yet developmental. She liked doing things together and having my undivided attention.

Sensory Integration Changes Are Lifelong

We brought Robin's OT/SI swing with us to Florida and hung it up in the middle of the garage, when needed. In those days, this was our lifeline to calm her behaviors. If she became anxious and frustrated, we'd say to her, "Let's go spin." It helped put her brain back on track. At twenty-six years old, we were still spinning as a last resort to correct behaviors.

One morning Robin was very frustrated because we were expecting houseguests. This was a change in routine. We didn't want to deal with her behavior when they arrived, so I said, "Let's go spin." Bob took Robin out to the garage to spin. After spinning and swinging, she came in, sat at the kitchen table, and started reading the newspaper. I noticed that she seemed confused. I asked what's wrong, and she said, "I'm dizzy." Bob and I laughed and gave her a big bear hug. This was the first time she'd been dizzy after spinning, which is a normal reaction and an OT/SI goal. Robin's behavior was appropriate when our guests arrived, and we retired the swing shortly thereafter.

We were never successful with animals in the house when Robin was younger. They either stayed under the bed in fear of her or they took on her personality. As an adult, she was ready for the relationship and the responsibility. Robin's cat, Snowball, has made a tremendous difference in her tactile needs. Robin receives gratification from Snowball every time she picks her up, and she is proud when Snowball purrs. Robin is responsible for another life, even if it's a cat. She talks to Snowball and Snowball is always available—Robin loves that! Snowball is her baby, a normal type of relationship for many people without autism.

Human touch and intimacy are important for everyone, including people with autism. When Robin was little, I used to lightly rub her back or just touch her hand—trying to get her to accept touching. She never reciprocated with the same gentle touch. Today, when Robin visits, I make a genuine effort to hug her hello or good-bye. Sometimes we sit as we did years ago for a few minutes. I will touch her hand or put my arm around her. I don't make a big deal out of it, but I do think it's important. In the last couple of years she has finally begun reciprocating with the same gentle touch.

Professionals often advocate that intimacy issues can directly relate to anxiety and frustration in people with autism. They think sexual satisfaction is the problem and many will even recommend a sex therapist to assist in this goal. It certainly would be an easy solution. Fortunately for Robin, I understand that touching does not have to mean sexual touch. We have discussed sexual relationships many times, and Robin seems comfortable as an independent single woman. Perhaps in time—

Chapter 4:
Speech and Language Therapy

Robin never babbled at all when she was a baby. We knew she had a voice, because she screamed very well—all the time in fact. We just weren't sure she could hear herself screaming.

Speech wasn't our biggest concern. We were much more concerned about her lack of awareness to anything or anyone in her environment. As a baby, we couldn't *see* her trying to think or use her brain.

My home program, when Robin attended Muriel Humphrey School for Retarded Children, helped me understand that communication involves much more than words. At home, I concentrated on presenting both verbal and non-verbal communication. If Robin could show me what she wanted, perhaps she wouldn't be so frustrated. As an example, I would say "juice?" Then I'd take her hand and we'd go to the refrigerator together, and I'd say "juice" again. I would then open the door and say the word "juice" again as I took the juice out of the refrigerator. Then, I would pour the juice in a glass and once more say the word "juice." My goal was for Robin to stand at the refrigerator, which would tell me she wanted some juice. Her next goal, hopefully, would be standing at the refrigerator as she said the word "juice."

This phase took a long time, but by the time Robin was five years old she was producing one- or two-word utterances with intent. At first, I kept my sentences simple ("Outside?") then added complexity later ("Want outside?" and later, "Do you want to go outside?"). As with all of Robin's learning, cooperation and participation depended on whether she was having a good day.

When Robin entered the public school system, it didn't appear to me that the programs and services were in any way coordinated. Her speech therapy was fifteen minutes twice a week, eventually progressing to group therapy once a week. It took Robin fifteen minutes just to get to the therapy room. By the time she had settled in the chair, it was time to go back to the classroom. Furthermore, there was no coordination between home learning and school learning. School notes home only reflected whether she'd had a good day or a bad day, not what skills she was working on and how to carry over the learning at home.

The Role of Speech-Language Therapy

In the 1970s in much of the country, speech therapy in the public school system focused on improving articulation and decreasing stuttering and voice problems. Today, the service may still be referred to as speech therapy, but it encompasses so much more. Speech therapy in the school setting is now separated into speech therapy, which addresses articulation and speech production, and language therapy, which addresses disorders associated with the comprehension and production of spoken and written language. Language therapy also focuses on the pragmatic or social use of language and it covers reading and written language. In some school districts, speech pathologists also do oral motor or feeding therapy.

Speech-language therapy (SLT) is provided by an individual licensed as a speech-language pathologist (SLP). The terms speech therapist, speech-language therapist and speech-language pathologist are generally considered interchangeable. Parents are not always aware of the significance of this therapy for individuals with developmental disabilities and how important it is to find the right therapist.

LorRainne Jones, MA, CCC-SLP, PhD

Understanding the Importance of Language Therapy

When Robin was ten years old, Bob and I agreed we needed to find help for her outside the public school system. Robin's private evaluations said she needed intense speech-language therapy, and we were put in touch with a SLT, Lesa Shelton.

Lesa said Robin's behaviors would improve when Robin learned to understand and use language appropriately. At this point, Robin's vocabulary was rote memorization of my words. Robin was not creating anything; she was mimicking me.

It was critical that I understood Robin's learning style if I was going to help her in our home program. One of the challenges for me was to understand all the professional terms used when trying to explain the challenges Robin was facing. I kept asking Lesa questions until I understood how Robin learned. Some of the terms included the following:

- *Receptive language, expressive language, and word retrieval:*

- ○ *Receptive* language is taking information *into* the brain. A person can hear and understand what someone is saying to them.
- ○ *Expressive* language is saying what you want to say, communicating. You are *expressing* yourself.
- ○ *Retrieval* is recalling information already stored in your brain and using it to express yourself. You are *retrieving* information from your memory bank.

- *Perseveration* is when a child asks or says the same thing over and over again and the answer is not registering with them to accept a person's response or answer.
- *Parallel* is a word often used to describe a person who doesn't socialize in social situations. It is often used to describe how young children play side by side but do not interact. They are *around* people but not communicating with them.
- *Echolalia* is when a person repeats another person's words, sentences, or questions verbatim rather than responding to the statement or question.
- *Splinter skills* can occur when a person has significant gaps in learning. You can be highly skilled at reading but have a tough time understanding language in general, including what you have read.
- *Figure-ground (attention and regulation):* This can include auditory and/or visual figure-ground discrimination. The child must be able to focus on the main *figure* or *signal* and not focus on the background.
  - ○ *Visual figure-ground discrimination*: Have you ever watched television and been distracted by glare on the screen from a light or sunny window in the room? This is how a person with visual figure-ground sees everything. Focusing on the main object (television) is very difficult.
  - ○ *Auditory figure-ground discrimination*: Another child talking softly in class will sound equal to the teacher's voice when both are talking at the same time.
- *Multi-sensory learners*: To understand or take information into a person's memory bank, some people need all learning channels to integrate information. There are three main channels of learning:

- ○ *Auditory learners* are good at understanding spoken language, understanding instructions from the teacher, and what a person is saying.
- ○ *Visual learners* take information into their brain through their visual system, which is their primary source of gaining information to which they can attach meaning. These people do better reading information, seeing it in print, or seeing an illustration.
- ○ *Tactile learners* are people who need to be physically involved in learning. They need to hold, move, and/or touch things to help the learning process.

Lesa, our speech-language therapist, really helped me to understand Robin for the first time. Robin could not take information into her brain, organize it so it made sense, and then respond to what she heard. Because of her figure-ground problems, anything in print had to be very basic. Too much on a page made focusing and attending difficult. Testing verified that Robin was a visual learner, even though she'd had two eye surgeries and didn't have twenty-twenty vision. In other words, Robin's primary sensory system for taking in and giving meaning to information was through her visual system (eyes), not her auditory system (ears).

The first priority for Lesa was to get Robin's attention so she could benefit from therapy. Lesa developed a structured, multi-sensory approach using behavior modification techniques that stressed positive reinforcement (see chapter 5: Behavior Interventions). She sat side by side with Robin and gave Robin her full attention during therapy sessions. She worked with Robin at Robin's pace, giving Robin time to process information and time to respond. Each session was one and a half hours long, twice a week. Robin did well with this approach and she understood what was expected of her. Every time Robin demonstrated the desired behavior, Lesa charted and posted it so Robin could see her progress. Robin liked the rewards. She liked the charts too—and there were so many charts. Robin enjoyed the charting and she eventually learned to chart herself.

Lesa taught language by teaching sentences of increasing length and complexity. To put sentences together, Robin had to learn vocabulary, pronunciation, spelling, definitions, and grammar rules. Lesa's approach was to teach Robin the responses to "wh" questions—*who, what, when, where, how, and why.* Verb tensing was taught. Lesa took the lead, and I supported her with our home school activities and materials that she approved.

Lesa was Robin's language therapist for over five years. When Robin returned to the public school system, she understood and could express her basic needs in complete sentences. She enjoyed reading and she was independently writing book reports with a structured outline. If Robin couldn't verbally communicate because she was frustrated, I'd give her paper and pencil, then ask her to put it in writing. Sometimes, that was easier for her.

When Robin returned to public school at sixteen years old, their therapist followed Lesa's program as best they could. I remember a conversation with Mrs. Billings, Robin's language therapist, during Robin's last year in high school. Robin still couldn't independently say a three-syllable word. She could sound them out when reading, but she couldn't pull them out of her brain (retrieve) much less use them independently in conversation. Robin was still very slow in processing language to answer anything. She understood more than she verbalized. I still found myself talking for Robin to make it easier so that she would not get frustrated.

It's Never Too Late: Adulthood

When Robin was twenty-four years old, her language skills seemed to be regressing. She could initiate simple questions, as needed, but any language was mostly confined to the home. Other people didn't understand the long lag time she needed to respond to their questions. She didn't initiate conversation and she definitely didn't add to conversation. She appeared social, but it was amazing how she didn't communicate in a social environment—unless she had a definite need. Interestingly enough, she had learned to look busy and show some appropriate body language.

Fortunately for Robin, the state of Florida had passed legislation that provided financial support to individuals with developmental disabilities so that they could continue to reside in their local communities. If Robin was going to have a full life in the community, she needed to be able to communicate comfortably with the people around her. That meant more speech therapy, with an emphasis on the acquisition of language skills.

Finding a licensed speech language pathologist for an adult isn't easy. Robin's first therapist in Florida came to our home twice a week for one-and-a-half-hour sessions. She was very good and patient with Robin. Eventually, a behavior therapist was added to the therapy sessions. They both went with Robin on outings in the community to encourage natural language experiences.

Robin's second therapist, Christine, came to her condominium twice a week for one-and-a-half-hour sessions. She worked tirelessly with Robin and was very successful. Because of the fragile transition to independent living,

Robin's behaviors were becoming a major concern. Christine developed charts and a behavior notebook, similar to what we'd done years ago, to help Robin through this transition. Unfortunately, Robin needed more consistency with this approach because of the many different people in her life.

LorRainne Jones, PhD, Kid Pro Therapy Services, was (and still is, at the time of this writing) Robin's third language therapist. Even though Robin was living in her own condominium, I wasn't ready to give up on her behavior and communication skills. She needed them now more than ever.

Interactive Metronome Therapy

After an initial evaluation, LorRainne recommended that Robin start with Interactive Metronome (IM) to help improve her auditory processing.[10] The IM literature states that individuals who participate in the IM program show improved processing abilities that affect attention and concentration, language processing, behavior (aggression and impulsivity), motor planning and sequencing, and academic performance. I agreed this is just what Robin needed.

IM is a computer program that challenges a person to match a computer-generated beat. It's a whole-body experience, using hands and feet. Robin hears a tone through headphones to a prescribed tempo, and she must match her movement to the tempo of the computer. If she's *too fast*, she gets a guide tone in one ear. If she's *too slow*, she receives a guide tone in the other ear. Robin has learned to use the guide tones, and this has increased the accuracy of her responses.

Half way through the ten-week IM program, I realized Robin was not engaging in verbal perseveration. She wasn't asking the same questions three or four times before accepting my answer. She didn't seem as anxious, and our conversations were more give-and-take. The rhythm of her conversation was natural. The second thing I noticed was that she had no scratch marks on her hands and arms from her cat. Robin always had scratches, even though Snowball had declawed front paws. Robin's reaction time upon realizing that the cat wanted to be put down improved dramatically. These two gains were huge for Robin.

Robin completed the IM ten-week program and within a three-month period her progress slowly began to fade. Scratches from the cat and perseveration returned. LorRainne started Robin on a second IM ten-week

---

10 www.interactivemetronome.com.

program. Robin quickly stabilized, but again she began to fade after about three months.

In spite of the difficulty maintaining gains, I was amazed at the progress Robin did make with IM. It was the first time I'd seen anything that improved her response delay that was so evident during conversation. I felt that maintaining this skill was crucial for Robin's employment opportunities.

To that end, for the next three years, IM was a regular part of Robin's language therapy program. We charted her self-best score, previous week's score, and the day's scores every week so Robin could see how she was progressing. IM is effective because it literally changes how the mind—and subsequently the body—responds to sound, and it measures these changes to the millisecond. It seems so very strenuous mentally and physically, I could never do IM week after week. I've asked Robin many times how she felt about doing it, thinking she might be bored with it. To my surprise, she always says she enjoys it. I have to believe her, because when Robin doesn't like something, she will let me know.

In the last four months, Robin has made major gains with her IM scores. They have improved to a level where she is within average range for her age. We have reduced IM to twice a month and we are carefully monitoring her scores. So far, so good. It's looking like we can go to once a month in the not-too-distant future.

Rhythmic Entrainment Intervention

LorRainne recommended Rhythmic Entrainment Intervention (REI), designed by Jeff Strong at the REI Institute, for Robin. REI is a twenty-minute music-and-rhythm auditory program specially designed for each individual. The REI Institute requires that each person complete a comprehensive intake form, which includes questions about specific things I never realized could be related. REI also considers the age of the individual when developing their program. The most frequently mentioned areas of improvements include attention and focus, energy levels, impulsivity, anxiety, mood, and sleep.

Admittedly, I was looking for help with Robin's obsessive issues. Robin listened to her CD daily for ten weeks as recommended by REI. I was impressed how relaxed she was at the end of the program. However, again, we began to see progress fade after a couple of months—and I saw no measurable improvement in her compulsive behaviors. When Jeff was notified, I filled out another intake form and he updated Robin's CD. She repeated the sessions for another ten weeks, as recommended. This time it worked. Robin graduated from the REI program. It was successful—her anxiety and frustrations are much more balanced, and her compulsive behaviors are much, much improved.[11]

Fast ForWord

Still hoping to improve Robin's reading and language understanding, we explored Fast ForWord, which utilizes a neuroscience approach to learning. The publisher of Fast ForWord, Scientific Learning, suggests that it combines the latest advances in brain research technology to develop learning and communication skills. Furthermore, students maintain the skills once they are mastered.[12] Robin used the interactive Fast ForWord software program for one hour, five days a week. The program improves language, reading, and comprehension. Robin uploaded her program data nightly to California so that LorRainne could monitor her progress.

This program concentrates on a variety of language and reading skills, skills that are important for Robin's continued success and independence. One example is sequencing paragraphs in order of importance. This has helped to improve Robin's communication, because she is more aware of the content and flow of information during conversations.

Relationship Development Intervention

Some time ago, LorRainne suggested that we consider the Relationship Development Intervention (RDI) program. She has been using RDI with families who have young children with autism, and she's been impressed with the gains she had seen. RDI is a guided participation program for parents to help their child with autism. It is developed by Steven E. Gutstein, PhD, of Sheely and Associates.[13]

Bob and I both realized that Robin's survival as an independent adult is due to her consistency, boundaries, structure, and repetition—her *static* brain. RDI has helped us realize Robin can get past the dependency limitations of a *static* brain and progress to a *dynamic brain*—resulting in flexible thinking, friendships, and shared experiences.

Robin definitely functions with a *static* brain. This is why she's successful as an independent person with autism. Anything or anyone breaking her

---

11   www.reiinstitute.com.

12   www.scilearn.com.

13   www.rdiconnect.com.

rules can potentially cause chaos, and Bob and I are the only ones who can successfully intervene. As examples:

- Recently Robin had a lead part in a play, and she depended on her notes far more than the director would have liked. I'd warned Robin that she needed to stop using them, but she didn't listen to me. During a subsequent practice, the director jerked the notes out of Robin's hand and jokingly said, "You don't need your notes anymore." Well, Robin gave the director her famous stare of anger and stomped off the set. She charged at me, saying, "I quit." It took me ten minutes to get Robin back under control and back on the set. The poor director was so confused. They had not seen the *true* Robin before. I'm just glad I was there to control the situation!

- People will ask Robin, "Where do you work?" Robin always answers, "Publix." They then ask, "How many hours do you work?" Robin gives a blank stare, because her hours change weekly. She could not give a flexible answer like, "I work *about* twenty hours a week." She also could not expand the question into an appropriate give-and-take conversation, much less add that she has two jobs.

RDI is a learning program, and Robin could never gain the skills it targets on her own. Her splintered skills and her *static* brain would have dominated her life forever, constantly necessitating support staff for her survival in the world around her.

Our family has been implementing the RDI program for two years now. LorRainne has been able to keep the therapy sessions and cost realistic for our family. Robin is fortunate, because as an independent adult she has many opportunities to incorporate RDI objectives into her daily life. She's moving through the program and is now in stage seven, with five stages to go. We have seen her *static* brain dramatically changing more into a *dynamic* brain. We see many examples of this every day:

- She is comfortable using gestures and facial expressions as she talks.
- She comfortably initiates conversation with others, not just her parents.
- She monitors others during conversations.
- She laughs at her mistakes and appropriately at the mistakes of others.

- She asks the other person for information to understand a shared experience.
- She is learning to feel comfortable telling jokes.
- She recognizes, understands, and uses four different degrees within each feeling.

She Needed It All

Everything Robin has had in language therapy helped her to get to where she is today. She has had a coordinated program that meets her needs. Her speech therapy at two years old laid the groundwork for Lesa to begin language therapy at ten years old. Even though Robin regressed in language skills after high school, starting again at twenty-eight years old has helped her move into successful independent community living.

There are likely many other programs in the developmental stages today designed to help people with autism. I hope so. The latest, most innovative programs will never be a substitute for the long hours required for therapy; however, for Robin, their timing has been perfect.

Chapter 5:
Behavior Interventions

"Inappropriate behavior is unacceptable in society."

Appropriate behaviors didn't happen automatically for Robin. Every appropriate behavior had to be carefully taught because she could not learn from consequences. She couldn't read a person's body language or facial expressions, much less understand what they were saying. As she became an adult, it was even more difficult for her to understand the difference between being *cute* and people *laughing* at her. How could she understand something was appropriate in one instance and not at others? Fortunately for Robin, she is a very sweet young lady. With family support, biomedical interventions, and therapies, she has been able to integrate *learned* appropriate behaviors into her adulthood.

When Robin was a child and confined to her *own little world*, professionals helped us understand that we needed to bring her into *our world*. That meant managing her behavior. We learned this was possible as long as we controlled her thought processes with boundaries, consistency, and structure. This guidance gave us the footing to keep moving forward as determined parents.

Key Components to Address Behaviors

- *Structure*: Robin needed things around her to be routine. Boundaries were her survival. Even though she couldn't tell time, meals needed to be at the same time every day. The simple act of going to bed and waking up at the same time was important. If Robin couldn't express herself with language, we realized, lack of structure was enough to encourage a tantrum or frustration in her behavior.

- *Consistency*: This is not the same as structure. Consistency for Robin was all about *me, my* behavior. I couldn't scream at her one minute when she was running and ignore it the next. If

I wanted to see progress in her, this was way too confusing. I couldn't say, "We're going to the store after you finish this workbook," lose track of time, and change my mind and not go. I had to be very careful what I promised. Consistency, not flexibility, in Robin's routine was progress for her.

- *Positive behavior modification*: I had to remember to catch Robin doing something right and reward positive behavior, instead of screaming and demanding compliance when she did something wrong. I couldn't use the same stand-by behavior techniques with Robin as I did with Pam and Karen. Timeout didn't work by itself, and neither did threatening or loud demanding of compliance, although I wasn't immune to this behavior at times. I was good at counting to three and reacting with appropriate and consistent follow-through *every time*. Verbal encouragement and praise with charts, stickers, rewards, and graphs are examples of success, but my consistency with all these techniques is what made it work.
- *Multi-sensory stimulation (sight, sound, touch)*: Robin couldn't take information into her brain through a single source, including behavior. It had to be all of her senses at the same time— touching it, hearing it, and seeing it. Blocks, pictures, flash cards—whatever added to the experience was a benefit. Even my primitive stick figures worked. It didn't have to be perfect, just multi-sensory stimulation. The more we did the better.

The Interconnection of Therapies

Learning for Robin was like an orchestra without a woodwind section. An orchestra needs all the instruments to be an orchestra. The same applies to Robin. Addressing her behavior but not her language and communication, or addressing her education, but not occupational therapy sensory integration, would fail to provide her with an appropriate education. Robin didn't need one thing—she needed it all! And she needed it all to work like an orchestra in order to realize a benefit.

School psychologists knew the importance of Robin receiving the appropriate support for her educational development. They emphasized it time after time, but there was no mechanism to make it happen. For example:

School psychologist, Robin 5 years old

"Robin seems to depend totally on external sources for whatever controls she uses and does not seem capable of functioning independently. She functions best in a highly structured situation with consistent behavior modification."

School psychologist, Robin 10 years old

"Robin needs a multi-sensory approach with a great deal of drill and reinforcement."

School psychologist, Robin 15 years old

"Robin requires considerable support and encouragement. She frustrates easily, becomes easily discouraged, and then withdraws unless she feels supported."

One public school administrator criticized the recommendations for Robin's program to include consistent behavior modification. He did not agree the public school system should reward positive behavior when teaching her. I looked at him puzzled and said, "Do you get a paycheck?" He did not respond. I said, "Your paycheck is your reward for doing a good job every day. What is the difference with Robin?"

Using Positive Behavior Modification Charts

Robin started private Language Therapy when she was ten years old, and the following year I started home schooling. Lesa Shelton, MS, CCC-SP, taught Robin language through positive behavior modification. Before academic learning could take place, Robin had to learn to sit still in a chair, listen, and pay attention. I reinforced Lesa's approach at home. It was up to me to reward positive behaviors instead of disciplining when Robin did something wrong. I had total confidence in Lesa's approach. I too had good days and bad days, but I tried to follow Lesa's plan.

I used charting for everything—except academics. I never charted grades, because Robin associated grades with failure in school. Grades were not my goal. My goal for Robin was positive behaviors and language skills. I charted activities anywhere in the house. It could be sitting at the table, standing, or working on the floor. I did not chart when we were out of the house (shopping, car rides, visiting friends, etc.).

Lesa helped me make a list of behaviors I needed to address for Robin. I picked one at a time from the list and didn't proceed to the next behavior until I had 50 percent success on what I was working on. I made a big deal out of the checkmarks or happy faces on the chart and they *were* Robin's reward.

It was important I used the same behavior goal for each assignment or activity—just a different chart on a different piece of paper. I was careful the assignment was not too complicated or had too much on a page or was too long.

All charts went on the refrigerator. Robin had a lot of charts. She shared her charts with Dad and Lesa. These charts were something multi-sensory she could show off with pride. She was very proud of her charts and she knew exactly what she did for each one. She learned to replace them on the refrigerator with new ones and she carefully filed the old ones in a folder. Yes, Robin was very chart focused!

Chart 1: Good Behavior

Goal: Sit at the table, pay attention to the teacher and use appropriate behavior.
Method: I showed her it was important to keep her feet on the floor while doing schoolwork. While she was working, I ignored her fidgeting feet but *caught* the moment her feet were not fidgeting. I said, "Good, you kept your feet on the floor" while I put a checkmark on the chart. This was done immediately while she was working, and she continued the assignment.

When I was satisfied with the behavior, I begin to eliminate the sentence and just said one word: "Good." Again, when I was satisfied with the behavior, I eliminated the verbal distraction "good" and just checked the chart. If needed, sometimes I would tap the chart with my pencil so she would refocus on the behavior that was expected of her.

After each assignment, we immediately counted the number of check marks on Chart 1 and bar graphed them in different colors on another chart, Chart 2. This chart helped Robin see how well she did from one day to another. As I added skills, I counted totals, which gave the appearance of greater success. Robin liked coloring the bar a different color each day.

Chart 1: Good Behavior

Feet on floor	✓✓✓✓
Hands to face	
Fidget with fingers	
Shoulder shrugs	

Mumbling
Exaggerated body movements
Eye contact
Smiling
Touching

Chart 2: Daily Graph

Daily Graph												
Date	1	2	3	4	5	6	7	8	9		1	1	1
April 26													
April 27													
April 28													
April 29													

I impressed myself with my ability to help Robin by charting at home. This was exactly what she needed. Charts helped Robin learn to focus and recognize appropriate body movements. When necessary, I could easily pull these basic behavior charts back into our program to address a specific behavior problem—which I often did!

Now that I had some short of attention and structure for Robin, Lesa had me tackle the language skills themselves. Again, we kept it visually simple. Robin loved workbooks. Workbooks are very visual, so I could easily use a multi-sensory approach to her learning with them. Again, I started with one positive verbal expectation from her at a time.

Chart 3: Positive Language

Goal: Using your brain and controlling your emotions during academic assignments.

Method: Same method as for Chart 1. I needed verbal answers to the questions I asked, not just pointing or otherwise showing me. Looking at the workbook page, I would say, "What is she holding in her hand?" Robin was expected to say, "Pencil." I immediately reinforced by saying, "Good telling me the answer" as I put a checkmark on the chart. After some success charting one language expectation, I added another to the chart and then another. Again, we totaled the checks and graphed the progress on a different chart.

POSITIVE LANGUAGE - USING YOUR BRAIN					Date:				
1. Good telling									
2. Good controlling your frustration									
3. Good additional information									
4. Good staying on task									
5. Good flexibility						·			
6. Good question									
Totals									

As time went on, Robin and I would expand and rearrange our charting methods. Learning this kind of flexibility was part of the experience. It was important to keep prompting her to leave her comfort zone.

While I was stabilizing my charting, Lesa continued expanding Robin's goals. Robin was very slow at processing her language to come up with a response. Lesa charted conversations in therapy as follows:

"I" for saying something *independently,*
"P" for saying something with *prompting,* and
"—" for saying something *incorrectly*

As always, they would count the marks after each session and graph by color on another chart (Robin never/seldom got "—").

For more efficiency and variety at home, after charting was well stabilized, I substituted the checkmarks on a chart with a click, using a clicker like the ones used to count people at events. At the end of the assignment (as we did with math or reading), I wrote the number of clicks counted by the clicker, and Robin charted them on a graph. It was amazing how the noise of the clicks seemed to stabilize Robin rather than distract her. As time went on, if I was not clicking, and the behavior was appropriate, Robin took the lead and said to me, "You forgot to click."

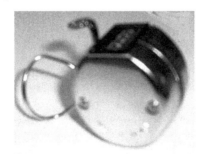

Fig. 5.1. Robin liked the reinforcement of the clicker.

The clicker, I found, is useful for behavior modification beyond those with autism. Recently my perfect seven-year-old grandson was visiting. I'm rather competitive at playing games, and he'd get frustrated if he lost, even crying. I found an old clicker, gave it to him, and told him to click when frustrated instead of crying. He did it! I was amazed he recognized his inappropriate behavior and could transfer it to the clicker so fast. We all began asking him to borrow the clicker if we were frustrated with the game. He took the clicker home.

Teaching Lifestyle Behaviors

Negotiating the Special Education Maze, by Winifred Anderson, Stephen Chitwood, Deidre Hayden, and Cherie Takemoto (Woodbine House, 1979-2008), offers more in their book than learning about special education laws and working with the school system. This book helped me learn how to identify and understand targeting specific behavior goals for Robin.

Before tackling any behavior change, they recommend using their "Parent Observation Record." Using this observation chart, taking notes and focusing on watching Robin's behavior in a specific situation helped me understand the *whys* and *hows* of exactly what needed to be changed. The reasons may not be as they appear.

After my observation, I adapted their "Developmental Achievement Chart" to my own specifications for Robin. By doing this, I kept the focus on Robin. Needless to say, I didn't always accomplish all these goals in the six-month timeframe. Many of my goals were suggested by Robin's therapists.

Robin's Developmental Achievement Goals Date:			
	CAN DO	WORKING ON	ACCOMPLISH WITHIN 6 MO.
MOVEMENT	Runs away outside and laughing	Walking side-by- side when shopping	Walking 50% of the time beside me without running
COMMUNICATION	Knows 20 words	Increase to 25 words	Focus on 5 words and use multi-sensory daily
SOCIALIZATION	Kicks sisters when they are on the floor	Sisters ask for a hug when she comes near them	Robin stops kicking her sisters
INDEPENDENCE	1 ½ hrs getting ready for school	Getting ready for school without an uproar in 1 hr	Have Robin chart steps for morning routine and when complete put on refrigerator
BALANCE	Body roll on the floor	Stay in a straight line when rolling	As a game, practice 3 x's a week rolling on the floor
THINKING SKILLS	Use 4 pieces in the game Concentration	Play Concentration using 8 pieces	Play Concentration 3 x's a week before fixing dinner
BEHAVIOR	Sit at table for 5 minutes	Sit at table for 10 minutes	After 5 minutes change activity for last 5 minutes

After I identified the specific behavior I wanted to work on, I then created my own follow-through chart with specific goals and steps. Breaking down a goal helped me slow down and recognize the necessary steps for Robin to achieve the task. I didn't assume she could do anything independently. I stayed with Robin while accomplishing the goal, we talked through each step, and we charted each step immediately after it was completed. The chart and reward were equal to Robin.

	Home Plan Based on Observation	Date:	
PROBLEM	**PRESENT LEVEL**	**GOAL**	**HOW TO ACHIEVE**
Getting ready for school	Takes 1 ½ hours. She's spacey or fussing wasting time and playing	Get ready for school in 1 hour without an uproar	• Robin turns off her alarm clock • Use bathroom (chart each step) • Get dressed (clothes already laid out) • Make bed • Clean room • Eat breakfast • Mom fix hair • Use bathroom (chart each step)

When appropriate, I took these goals and made Robin her own chart so she could focus more on her independence. She would check off the assignment and receive stickers when completed appropriately. They, too, went on the refrigerator.

Garnering the Support of Adults, Not Peers

Robin's behaviors were confusing to her peers because of her erratic movements or her standoffishness, and I didn't blame them. She could not relate to them. If they asked her a question, she just *stared*. If Robin didn't say something, they were off on another subject before she spoke. I often felt if she just stuttered at least people would know she was trying to speak.

A *light bulb* moment for me was the realization that my goal for Robin was not her childhood peers. Yes, she needed their socialization to grow, but her peer relationships were never going to evolve into true friendships. My goal was adults. That's when peer relationships are really important for her and must happen—so I began focusing on adults.

Robin needed to feel accepted by people other than our family. Our extended family, neighbors, and friends had the patience to wait the long lag time for Robin to respond to a question. Our neighborhood social life revolved around backyard holiday picnics, birthday parties, and volleyball games. They usually included about ten families.

One of these families, the Sparks, moved back to the city. They spent many weekends (Friday night through Sunday afternoon) at our house with their young son. Robin had to learn she was not always the priority these weekends and she had to share. They were very patient with Robin and she eventually accepted them into her world. Robin benefited greatly from this change in her routine. So did I.

After Robin graduated from high school, Aunt Vera and Uncle Ford visited us every Sunday afternoon. Aunt Vera had recently been hospitalized with a stroke, and she used a wheelchair. Robin always entertained Aunt Vera because I had to fix dinner. Robin loved visiting and taking care of her needs. They'd sit and talk, looking out the sliding glass door, as Uncle Ford and Bob worked at the barn for several hours—every Sunday afternoon.

Understanding that Modification Takes Time

I believe behavior is much more than being taught the difference between right and wrong. Success includes being appropriate and a part of the world around you. The following are examples of behaviors:

- Compassion for others
- Self-awareness (clothes, hygiene, hair, etc.)
- Health and safety
- Smiling, eye contact, and appropriate communication skills
- Independence, responsibility, assertiveness, and confidence
- Appropriateness in the community

I attended a presentation telling parents that we are too impatient and expect immediate changes in behaviors previously learned by our children. The presenter stressed that parents give up too soon on their children. She knew the disability population well and told us some behavior changes can take three to five years to integrate as learned skills.

At first I disagreed with her, but as Robin grew into adulthood, I really recognized this challenge. I was ready for Robin's independence, but Robin was not ready to be independent. She wanted it, but wanting and achieving are two different things.

It has taken Robin five years, with our support, to learn to be a competent and independent adult.

Chapter 6:
Socialization and Self-Image

I had to be creative and make meaningful socialization opportunities happen for Robin in her childhood. I did not expect them to be handed to me on a silver platter. Knowing this, I continually felt defeated when she was a child. I really did try, but Robin could not remain focused on any activity. She didn't relate to the other children. She didn't care. She didn't fit in. So I stopped making her socialization my priority.

All that changed when she was ten years old. Robin's psychologist, Edwin Carter, PhD, shamed me into once again making Robin's socialization my priority. To make his point, Dr. Carter asked me what the logo was on a boy's shirt as we walked into his waiting room. I, of course, didn't know. He told me Robin needed to know these things, since they were age appropriate. It was a screen print of R2-D2, the *Star Wars* character. He made his point—lesson learned! Dr. Carter became my guide for the next five years.

Preparing for Positive Socialization Experiences

From past experience, I knew plopping Robin into any social situation didn't benefit her or others. I decided to step back from the disability community and work with parents of typical children. They needed to feel Robin was a good example for their child and that she deserved the same opportunities to benefit from an activity as their child. I felt that:

- Typical children should not be expected to continually make allowances for Robin's inappropriate behaviors; and
- Typical children should not be limited in an activity just because Robin was a part of the group.

Robin needed preparation. Her behavior needed to be appropriate, and she needed to like the social activity. Only then, I felt, she would be accepted by her peers. She needed to feel safe and she needed to look appropriate to have a positive self-image. Thus, the first year of home schooling, I challenged Robin by expanding her tolerance limits until she could respond appropriately and act appropriately outside her given boundaries (see chapter 5: Behavior Interventions).

Finding and Creating Socialization in Childhood

I kept my eyes and ears wide open looking for social opportunities for Robin. I didn't have anything in mind, except that it needed to be a positive experience for her. I searched our local small-town newspaper, with three requirements in mind:

1. It needed to be something where she could feel successful.
2. It needed to be long-term.
3. I needed to be involved.

There was an announcement in our local newspaper that new baton classes were starting up for the White Star Majorette Corps. In Virginia, there were lots of local firemen and holiday parades. The corps member ages were three to twenty-two years old, and they often reached eighty twirlers.

Bob took Robin to the advertised practice night. I thought, if a three year old could twirl a baton, so could Robin! Kitty Baugh, the director, called me the following morning and said, "I thought she had autism?" I told her yes, but I felt she could handle Robin in her classes if I also attended. Kitty agreed to accept the challenge. To reinforce the weekly lessons, Robin also had weekly private lessons to help her keep up with the class. I knew Kitty's reputation well, and I had confidence in our relationship.

Kitty took it slow and positive. First, she taught Robin very basic rhythm and marching skills, and Robin learned to carry the main corps banner, along with another girl, down the middle of the street. Next, Robin carried a squad banner by herself—again down the middle of the street. Robin had to learn it was important the banner wasn't too far ahead or too far behind. Banner carriers wore white pants and a red shirt with white tennis shoes. Robin was proud of her uniform.

Robin and I practiced her batons daily and she took her weekly lessons seriously. She wanted to twirl. As time went by, with weekly group lessons and private lessons, Robin officially started twirling one baton with a younger age group squad. For this, she got the full majorette uniform—a red sequin top, short white skirt, boots, and a hat. She was smiling from ear to ear, clearly very proud of herself.

Twirling with Robin's age group was the next priority, but Robin wasn't ready to twirl two batons in a parade. Therefore, Kitty developed another temporary goal for Robin. She designed a solo flag routine specifically for Robin so she could be in her peer squad.

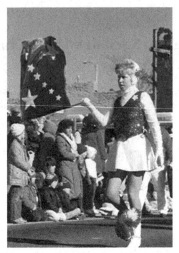

Fig. 6.1. Robin doing her flag routine in a local parade.

The following year, Robin reached her goal and began twirling two batons with her age group. This was an incredible day! This is the same child who couldn't *cross midline* (one hand over the other) just six years before (see chapter 3: Occupational Therapy Sensory Integration). Now she was twirling two batons, going in separate directions, to a routine on a parade route.

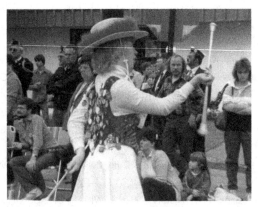

Fig. 6.2. Robin finally advanced to twirling two batons.

Robin was so excited and proud of herself when she became a White Star Majorette. The back of uniform was full of first, second, and third-place competition ribbons given by the judges from each parade. She was part of the team. Twirling didn't require language. No one cared about Robin's standoffishness as long as she could keep up with the squad, and she did. Parades were usually on Thursdays and Saturdays during season. I attended them all, and Bob attended when he was not on travel.

There was another notice in our local newspaper of a new 4-H club forming in our area. I knew nothing about 4-H, but I had been a Girl Scout. Living on a mini-farm with animals, 4-H sounded interesting.

After attending the meeting, I realized 4-H centered around three areas—leadership, citizenship, and life skills. I was excited, because Robin needed these goals for her daily living lessons in our home school. 4-H helped me emphasize a lifestyle of socialization in the community. The four leaves of the clover emblem stand for head, heart, hands, and health.

I cannot say enough good things about 4-H.[14] According to the 4-H Web site, today there are over seven million individuals in 4-H in the United States, making 4-H the largest out-of-school youth program. Ages vary among states, but most students can participate from eight to eighteen years old. 4-H is part of the Cooperative Extension System, a non-profit program operated through each state's land grant university.

Community projects and volunteering were part of Robin's 4-H experience. She learned the importance of giving to others. All of her projects included workbooks and competitive oral presentations. We developed and rehearsed her rote presentations, using three-by-five cards, as part of our home school. The Extension Office rewarded local and state presentations and project books with ribbons and certificates. They went on Robin's bedroom wall, where they remained as positive reinforcements.

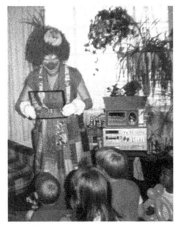

Fig. 6.3. Robin as Silly Sarah performing her magic tricks.

---

14 www.4-H.org.

Robin's 4-H club held regular weekly meetings, led by its membership. These meetings were governed by protocols known as *Robert's Rules of Order*. They elected officers and learned how to participate in an organization. The Extension Office personnel worked closely with the membership and adult advisors for reinforcement.

Club members chose which projects they wanted to work on. Most were done in small groups, and parents or local professionals led the selected projects. Robin's 4-H projects included citizenship, leadership, clowning, fundraising, poultry, nutrition, photography, health, creative writing, consumer, grandparents, cooking, and marine science.

Robin's talent for the annual 4-H talent show was baton twirling. I made special outfits and Kitty taught Robin solo routines to popular music. Many routines included dimming the house lights and using special light sticks on the ends of her batons. Robin worked hard on these performances and she received a lot of encouragement from her peers to perform on such a big stage by herself.

Many of the 4-H members submitted items for judging at the county fair. The members planned and strategized what to enter. Crafts were very difficult for Robin, but she wanted to be included as part of the group, so she did them.

Leadership, citizenship, and life skills are exactly what Robin needed. Robin was in 4-H for seven years and she is a 4-H All Star (similar to an Eagle Scout in Boy Scouts).

Finding and Creating Socialization in Adulthood

After moving to Florida when Robin was twenty-two years old, we started shopping around for socialization and community activities. She had talked about taking martial arts for years and this is where we started.

Robin took pre-GED classes for awhile, but they required a lot of independent study and self-motivation. I actually thought about taking them with her, but I felt she was too old for her mother's support in a classroom. Robin and I went to the library and reviewed the GED curriculum. We both agreed she did not need her GED.

Just because Robin was not successful with mainstream adult academic classes, that didn't mean she couldn't learn. Education was social involvement with other people, and social involvement was more important than academics.

Robin joined our church's adult choir and enjoyed singing and forming relationships with other choir members. She's a natural alto, and really likes music. Taking a cue from Robin's dedication to the choir, we asked the pianist if she gave lessons. She did. Robin bought an electric piano, and Suzanne became Robin's piano teacher for over two years, involving her in a number of recitals. Piano lessons were excellent for Robin, and I was amazed she could learn to read music *and* play the piano at the same time. Suzanne was very patient, particularly as I observed some of Robin's inappropriate behaviors during their lessons.

At this point I was attacking socialization with a band-aid, and much more was needed. To make genuine friendships, Robin needed a lot of constant social opportunities with other people. I had to find natural opportunities where friendships could develop and expand. In today's society, that is not easy.

Kristine and Robin were in the same adult Sunday school class at our church. They were acquaintances, not friends. Kristine had just graduated from St. Petersburg Junior College, and her mother, Denice, asked me if Robin would like to be Kristine's roommate. I said, "Robin needs a friend first. Let me tell you my idea." We wrote a mission statement and Mainstreamed Adult Singles at Home (MASH) was born.

MASH's Mission Statement:

"MASH encourages and supports *challenged* adults to meet and socialize with their peers and to experience the enjoyment of friendship, fun, and social events. Emphasis is placed on single adults living at home with parents or relatives who have goals to expand beyond the home and function in the community. Challenged young adults are individuals who do not easily interact or are accepted by their peers because of shyness, phobias, insecurities, or other social issues. This includes being mentally and physically disabled."

Denice and I became a team. We advertised in local newspapers and people came. If a MASH member didn't drive, their parents were responsible for transportation. MASH was not free. Part of learning responsibility in life is to pay your own way to activities or events. Life is hard sometimes, a reality that helped to keep the membership to around twenty members.

Parents of MASH members knew what their young adults needed most. We wanted to *own* the program, not a government agency. We decided to spend our energies on the MASH members, not incorporating or organizing a non-profit organization. We weren't interested in a paid administrator or grants for our survival. We all pitched in!

At first, we met monthly at our local McDonalds to plan activities—then we moved to a local church when we outgrew their space. One family started modeling classes for the girls, including fashion shows. Another organized local dinner and dancing cruises. Members attended professional sporting events, including football, baseball, and hockey games. Many of the MASH members planned bowling or movie nights. One of the parents organized an evening life skills class. Another found materials and a boat trailer for a Christmas parade float. Several MASH members had holiday parties in their home.

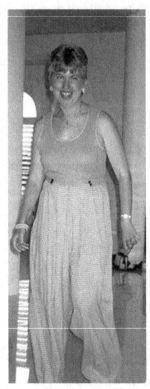

Fig. 6.4. Robin practicing for a MASH modeling show.

Members of MASH enjoyed opportunities never afforded them before. Developing friendships included talking on the telephone, making plans, and working together—not just monthly meetings. They had so many activities, some members learned to make choices for the first time. They learned from each other. Claudia was MASH's *social butterfly*, and she was a role model for Robin. Paul purchased a condominium and gave me the vision that Robin might be able to live on her own someday. Several of the members could drive, so why couldn't Robin? The same thing applied to employment. The members fed off each other. So did the parents.

MASH was growing, and everything was going well; however, we realized we really did need structure to secure our existence. Parents are dedicated and wonderful, but we wanted to make sure the organization lasted beyond any of the member or parents' commitments. We needed stability without incorporating.

We asked our local YMCA for membership scholarships for the MASH members and additional social activities. Doug, a sixteen-year-old high school student at the time, walked into the doorway where we were meeting and said, "I want to be part of this." To our advantage, Doug had lots of friends!

Young singles typically go out on Friday nights. Thus, the YMCA immediately started weekly Friday-night swimming socials for MASH. This gave MASH identity at the YMCA and thus the community.

One of the MASH parents was involved in Special Olympics. Doug and company took on Special Olympics as a volunteer project. MASH members practiced hard and developed a volleyball team. In the off-season of volleyball, swimming became a Special Olympic sport. Another parent started bocce ball, and another parent golf.

Yet another parent started the MASH Players and became the director of their annual performance. This is very serious and requires six weeks of practice. I was taking pictures at a final dress rehearsal one night when I turned from the stage and saw seven mothers, my friends, sitting at a rectangle table intently watching the performance. It brought tears to my eyes. We mothers never got to share these moments with our young adults when they were teenagers. Now we can. We're all such a positive support system for each other. These drama performances have a full house each year. Siblings schedule their Florida vacations so they can attend and share the experience as a family.

MASH members have four separate arms in our community: MASH Social Group (member/parent), MASH YMCA (no parents allowed), MASH Special Olympics, and MASH Players.

I stepped back from MASH after the first year, but Robin is still an active member. MASH is now fourteen years old. The YMCA leadership has passed to a new set of advisors, and the transition has been very successful. The MASH members renamed the group "Mainstreamed Adults Sharing Hope." The church where we hold our social group meetings is now sponsoring our volleyball team.

As MASH was forming, Robin and I joined our local Agency for Persons with Disabilities (APD) Family Care Council (FCC). FCC members are a gubernatorial appointment. I was interested in the council because it was something Robin and I could do together as equal adults. I thought it would also help her understand, learn, and respect the services she was receiving from state funding. Their legislated functions are to:

- *Assist* in providing information and outreach to families;
- *Review* the effectiveness of the developmental disabilities program;
- *Advise* administrators with respect to the community and family support system; and
- *Meet* and share information.

After attending the first FCC meeting, Robin and I almost didn't return. There was no organization and no program. In spite of this, Robin and I started volunteering. She was able to tap into her 4-H days with meeting protocols. She learned the importance of agendas, meeting responsibilities, and completing assignments.

Robin and I have traveled throughout Florida to various meetings, representing individuals with developmental disabilities and their families. We have attended trainings on *quality* services, abuse, guardianship, self-determination, employment, Social Security, and supported living. Robin has given a Microsoft PowerPoint presentation called *My Goals, My Dreams* at several conferences. She loves to talk about herself.

FCC is where Robin and I grew in our vision for her future. I was very impressed with other individuals on the council and their responsibilities and independence. Brian, Tyler, Sandy, Louise, and Ron were good examples of success; however, none of them had autism. Robin was on the council for six years. Since then she has stepped back from FCC. It was definitely time for us to go our separate ways, and it was a transition that came naturally.

Importance of Self: Self-image and Self-confidence

Many people with autism do not have a concept of self-image or self-confidence because they cannot connect with their feelings. Yet, feelings are critical on our journey in life—our *own* feelings as well as recognizing the feelings of others.

As a young child, Robin definitely didn't have an image of herself. Entering the school system, her negative experiences promoted failure after failure. When I began home schooling, we focused on successes in her life—no more failures. We didn't emphasize grades; rather, the focus was on positive behaviors and becoming a part of the world around her. To do this, we congratulated her, we watched her performances, we took lots of pictures, and we encouraged her abilities. Robin's bedroom walls were full of her ribbons, trophies, and other accolades as reminders of her achievements. Robin blossomed with this approach in spite of her autism. She was very proud of herself and she never hesitated sharing her rewards with family and friends.

All the tireless and carefully planned events in Robin's childhood paved the way for her continued socialization and employment as an adult. Her personality, compassion, self-image, confidence, and positive attitude are her rewards—along with the smile she wears on her face.

Chapter 7:
Education

Parents for compliance your faith has been torn.
You work for all children, not just your own.
Working within the system you've tried to improve
Education for the handicapped in our public schools.

Education is expensive,
Our children *can* learn.
They can become productive adults
And will, when education takes a turn.

All this Individual Education Planning in the IEP,
It's supposed to benefit our children appropriately.
Something is drastically happening within our schools
When the Feds allow the counties to break all the rules!

Look at our children,
See how they learn.
How I wish my county spent as much quality time teaching
As they do in bureaucratic paperwork preaching!

Our Federal government reviews bureaucratic paperwork.
They toil and our counties have learned to comply.
Pity the children's schoolwork
And the educational benefit the Feds were supposed to supply.

Parents for compliance you feel down-trodden and sore.
How do I know? I've been there before.
We need court action to prove we are right
These children are screaming for an education that's right!

A law isn't a law until it's been proven in court.
If I had $50,000, I'd take them to court.
I don't, however, so I teach my child at home
The child my county said is retarded is going to make it on her own!

Yes, our counties give teachers courses in paperwork and the law.
Oh, how I wish it were phonics and math that I saw.
To parents whose children are missing the boat
4-H has good programs, including self-image and hope!

—Ann Millan, 1983

The Problems of Public Schooling

Robin was not progressing in school. Every spring her school Individual Education Plan (IEP) meeting included a table full of professionals—and me. Every year I heard the same thing—she couldn't learn, she didn't fit in, she wasn't improving, she was a distraction to the class, and she needed a different school placement.

Following my instincts, I knew this was all wrong. Robin was staying in her *own little world* for them and she was not receiving an appropriate education. It took Robin's teachers until April every school year to understand how she learned. Every year, teachers would privately apologize to me as they passed the baton to another teacher in a different school with a different principal.

Robin was placed in a special education learning disability class when she was seven. I so wanted this placement to work for her. The teacher, Mrs. Hartley, was really good. She established Robin's basis for phonics and expected Robin to participate with the class. Robin really tried. As an example, Fridays were spelling test day. The test words this particular day were colors. Robin pulled out her box of crayons and copied each spelling word off the crayon wrapper as the words were called out to the class. Mrs. Hartley was shocked at Robin's creative initiative, and Robin got an "A" on the test!

However, Robin couldn't keep up with the pace of Mrs. Hartley's class. She had to teach to the whole class, not just to Robin's learning style. The following year, Robin was demoted back to a learning disability language delayed class at yet another school. This class, too, did not meet Robin's needs, and the following year the school system was planning another demotion to the special education building. In this placement she would not be around typical children, only children with severe disabilities.

Backed against a wall, we placed Robin back in the same private school she attended when she was five years old the following year—knowing we could only afford one year.

Home Schooling with Calvert

I purchased the third grade *Calvert Home School* curriculum.[15] It was way too difficult for Robin originally, but it was a very structured and workable program for me to follow. I could do this. The first year I hardly opened Calvert, because Robin needed preparation. I worked on behavior, attention span, frustration, anxiety, and therapies. We traveled to language therapy (see chapter 4: Speech and Language Therapy), psychological counseling (see chapter 6: Socialization and Self-Image), and art therapy. I had a home program for occupational therapy sensory integration (see chapter 3: Occupational Therapy Sensory Integration). This is the year I became proficient in charting (see chapter 5: Behavior Interventions). I learned to hold Robin's attention for twenty minutes at a time with one activity. She made tremendous progress.

The following year I took on the challenge of Calvert. Calvert gave the option of their staff grading quarterly tests. This removed me from that role. I could honestly say to Robin, "Calvert expects you to know this."

Before Robin woke each morning, I did my lesson planning. She started each day with the same routine—she ate breakfast, cleaned her room, dressed herself, and headed for the barn to let the chickens out and collect their eggs. Her official school day was non-stop, from ten to four.

I was amazed how she absorbed the educational information. I taught Calvert world history, U.S. history, geography, art, mythology, science, spelling, critical writing, reading, and math. She got it all! We were actually having fun.

Calvert was excellent and it gave me the necessary structure to be a teacher. It was easy to add additional materials for reinforcement of skills needed—particularly for math, reading, and comprehension.

Strengthening Reading Comprehension Skills

Mrs. Hartley was very helpful when I decided to home school Robin. She recommended a phonetic reading and workbook series she'd used in her classroom. In addition, I used *The Writing Road to Reading* (QUILL, Harper Resource, an imprint of Harper Collins Publishers, 1957-2003) by Romalda Bishop Spalding.[16] (I had taken the Spalding forty-hour teacher's instruction course several years earlier.)

---

15 www.calvertschool.org.
16 www.spalding.org.

Everything complemented Calvert. Spalding had a structured approach to cursive writing—cursive was much easier because of the flowing motion. Spalding discouraged guessing answers. If Robin hesitated too long or seemed confused with something, I told her the answer. I learned from a conference I'd attended that it was best to use yellow lined paper for children with visual problems and never glossy white paper, so I did.

As additional reinforcement, I used *Explode the Code*, a Systematic Sequential and Explicit Phonics Program by Nancy M. Hall.[17] Robin loved *Explode the Code*, and she learned to do the assignments independently. Each workbook was clear and simple. They approached the same phonetic assignment four different ways, and they designed their series for success. *Explode the Code* workbooks are still very popular and available today. They currently have twenty-one workbooks to encourage repetition and structured learning.

Many schools and workbooks use slash marks between syllables (a/chieve/ment). This was too confusing for Robin, who I believe mistook the slash marks for letters or numbers. With her behavior, visual, and intellectual problems, she could never get past the slash marks. For Robin, I used ocean-type waves to separate syllables *under* each word. If she hesitated with a word, I would draw wave lines under the word and then she would phonically sound it out. As time went on, if she had trouble sounding out a word, she would independently *wave* the syllables herself while reading.

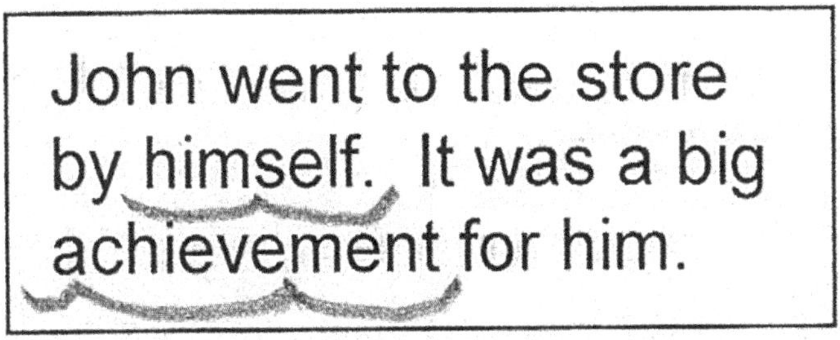

John went to the store by himself. It was a big achievement for him.

Fig. 7.1. How to *wave* syllables.

I always had a bright orange plastic strip (1″ x 4″) to slide down the page for smooth reading. This went *above* the line read, and I slowly moved it downward as she read. It was distracting, and limited her reading flow, to be directly *under* the actual line read or to use my finger. As time went on, I used a clicker to speed up her reading rhythm, continually clicking when she was reading correctly (see chapter 5: Behavior Interventions). This was

---

17   www.epsbooks.com.

amazingly successful, and the clicking sound didn't distract her. Interestingly, it helped keep her more focused. Robin took the leadership role in reading. We graphed the number of clicks daily and she focused on beating her best score, reading more independently and longer each day.

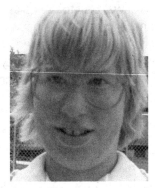

Fig. 7.2. Robin during her home school years.

Robin became a good speller. Bob made us colored wooden blocks. A green block (start) was the prefix, we used a blue block for each middle syllable, and a red block was the suffix or end (stop). As we sounded out spelling words, I hit the appropriate color block on the table, saying the sounds or word. Next, she would do it. We wrote the word and *waved* the syllables. We looked the words up in the dictionary together for definitions. We diagrammed sentences using *who, what, when, where, how* and then wrote a sentence.

Building Math Skills

Math was Robin's weakest subject. She had to learn math *place value*. To encourage multi-sensory thinking, I decided to use objects she could touch to understand—tens, hundreds, thousands, and millions. Plastic coffee stirrers were the cheapest objects I could find. She wrapped bundles of ten coffee stirrers each, with rubber bands, until we reached one million—one hundred thousand bundles of ten coffee stirrers each. They *overflowed* a laundry basket. We played with them, counted them, stacked them, and tested with them. She got it!

I carefully followed the developmental sequencing of Calvert's math book. We took our time, and I didn't go to the next lesson until I felt she grasped the current lesson. With addition, subtraction, multiplication, and division, I highlighted in green (go) where to start as a clue. I encouraged, and she relied heavily on, specialized cheat sheets. I always tried to remove every obstacle to accomplish the task. No need to rewrite the math problems—she wrote answers directly in her textbook. In Robin's Nest School, she only had to complete half the problems correctly on the page. Repetition of fifty problems was not necessary, but twenty-five correct answers were. Sometimes I'd *star* the problems I wanted her to do. Again, my goal was a positive math experience, not negative frustration and anxiousness.

Teaching Multiplication Tables

Robin knows her multiplication tables well. She knew the concept of "sets" from previous lessons. First, I explained it was easier and quicker to get a total by multiplying than adding. Using poker chips I had her count the chips, say fifteen of them. She counted them, and then I placed them on the kitchen table in "sets" of five and showed her 3 x 5 = 15.

To start teaching the tables, I then said, "If you have nothing, zero, and you multiply it by one, what do you have? You still have nothing, right?" I explained this many different ways. I reinforced with the flash cards (0 x 1 = 0, 0 x 2 = 0, 0 x 3 = 0, etc.). After Robin had acquired these concepts, I made the rest of the multiplication tables into a floor exercise.

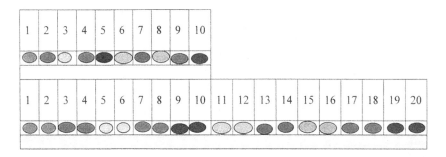

Fig. 7.3. Teaching multiplication tables.

To make this table, you will need:
1. 8.5" x 14" legal-size paper, turned sideways, with ten connecting squares drawn across the top, about 1" x 1".
2. 10 sets each of 10 jewels (craft store). Each set a different color.

Directions:

Only teach one table at a time until learned.
- Learning 1s tables — 10 different colors of 1 each
- Learning 2s tables — 10 different colors of 2 each
- Learning 3s tables — 10 different colors of 3 each
- Etc.

I taught one table on the chart at a time. After Robin put the jewels on the table being learned, we then reinforced the lesson using flash cards and laid out sets of poker chips. I then went to the next table. As the table numbers grew, we had to keep taping additional legal-size papers to the chart length. This chart was about 6 feet long when completed. When she knew her multiplication tables well, I then reversed the concept so she could learn to divide.

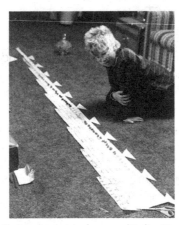

Fig. 7.4. Robin learning her multiplication tables.

Robin loved working with objects. Originally, I worried she would have problems with certain calculations (e.g., 8 x 3 = 24 and 6 x 4 = 24), but that never bothered her, because she got the concept. Later, if needed, she had a small laminated paper multiplication table available at all times. She stopped using the table because it was slowing her down for answers. She proofed her own work using a calculator.

Mapping Out Science, History, and Geography

Robin took all the typical subjects learned in school by typical children, and I was amazed at the difference this made in her psychological evaluations.

Most importantly, I made a timeline and strung it down our family room wall to help clarify time and space. To help Robin understand the BC/ AD dating system, I made five-by-eight cards; BC dates were green and AD dates were red until 1776—then I added a blue border on the red cards to emphasize the beginning of the United States. I had a card for every hundred years.

We punched a hole in each card at the center top and arranged them on a rope in order. On the bottom of each card, we punched another hole in the center to attach everything on that specific card as we studied it. We used an opened paper clip as a hanger. The wall was full of cards, and we often had to play detective to find the right card for the lesson. The timeline was a mess with all the things hanging below it, but Robin didn't care. It was great and helped her see how much we had learned.

To get her started using the timeline, we studied the presidents of the United States and put each on the timeline. I found a tourist booklet with each president on a separate page and their bios on the back of the page. We tore these out, read the bios, and placed them on the timeline. This helped Robin see how young our country was in relation to the whole world. If we had questions, we went to the encyclopedias or dictionary. I had a world globe and we referred to it often. We then researched and found related pictures: the Statue of Liberty, the Washington Monument, national parks, etc.

To reinforce her reading level, we used stories from Calvert about the fall of the Roman Empire, Alexander the Great, King Arthur, and Robinson Crusoe. She also learned the difference between political systems—communism, capitalism, and socialism.

I purchased test tubes and we did all the experiments in our science books. Many of these were very time consuming, but fun. We made our own mobile of the solar system to help her understand that planets revolve around the sun, not the other way around.

Geography books helped to define the seasons. We included stories about different terrains and foods produced in different regions. Maps reinforced different countries, states, and capitals. Other maps were more localized to specific communities and the assignment was how to get from one place to another in our community.

Developing Life Skills

Since I was the teacher, I could pick and choose life-skill activities I felt Robin needed to learn.

- *Typing skills*: The Commodore VIC 20 computer was the first affordable home computer available in the early 1980s. I purchased an excellent typing program, and Robin learned to type. I have yet to find a comparable typing program for IBM or Mac today. She practiced daily.
- *Socialization*: I had a full-length mirror on the family room wall, with easel paper taped down one side holding Robin's baton

routine instructions. Robin memorized the routines. She loved all her 4-H project workbooks, and they complemented her English and writing lessons. 4-H also provided the audience for her rote presentations (see chapter 6: Socialization and Self-Image).

- *Games*: Robin and I spent many hours playing Canasta, a two-player game. I was told to play games and do puzzles that encouraged reasoning skills not rote memorization. We could stop and start any time and continue finishing later. Yes, we kept score!

- *Responsibilities*: Robin was responsible for the chickens. She collected all the eggs, counted them, and sold them to friends and neighbors. We had a riding lawnmower, and Bob supervised as she mowed the grass. Eventually Bob gave her driving lessons in the local high school parking lot on weekends, and she passed her Virginia State learner's permit test. Robin was a good driver in the parking lot but afraid to drive on the street. (Interestingly, this experience probably laid the groundwork for Robin's desire to drive at thirty years old.)

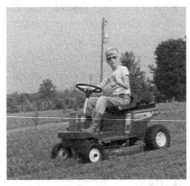

Fig. 7.5. Mowing the lawn fueled our vision for driving a car.

Many of Robin's educational and daily living assignments were coordinated with her therapies and school program. Teaching all the structured lessons, I was very aware of weaknesses in my program that needed to be addressed. For example:

- *Scissors*: Strength, attention span, eye-hand coordination, and motivation are all required to use scissors. This was very hard for Robin, even at twelve years old. I used coupons from the weekly Sunday newspaper. Robin learned to cut out coupons, realizing they were items she wanted. As the years passed, she learned to purge the outdated coupons. She cut them all out and filed them in a box. She still does this today.

- *Cooking*: I had Robin make a macaroni-and-cheese casserole from a boxed mix. She did all the steps as we read the instructions, and we talked them through, *except* that I poured the pot of boiling noodles in the strainer at the sink. After we finished, I had Robin write a paper on "How to Make Macaroni and Cheese." She did an excellent job, including all the steps *she* had performed, leaving out what I did. (This assignment emphasized to me the importance of multi-sensory input and of Robin doing each step.)

Calvert is a regular school program, not a special education curriculum. Fortunately, they didn't require each grade to be completed in a single year. Robin took two years for each grade. She received a promotion certificate for third, fourth, and fifth grade. The font size of the sixth-grade material was smaller, and the curriculum was becoming too difficult. Robin wanted to attend public school and graduate—she wanted the cap-and-gown experience. It was a good excuse to stop.

Robin went from testing at the prekindergarten level or lower in the public school system to testing at sixth-grade level in five years of home schooling. Her General Information score on educational testing was at the tenth-grade level.

Returning to Public School and Walking for Graduation

Robin returned to the public school system for her last two years of high school. She knew a lot of the students through 4-H and majorettes. The first year she attended half day, receiving language therapy, learning disabilities (LD) class, and employment class. The LD teacher gave Robin one-on-one instruction for the Virginia Tenth Grade State Competency Test. Robin passed both tests—reading and math. Robin's employment class teacher found her a volunteer position at our local community mini-library. Robin scanned every library book into a computer program for their inventory. Robin's language therapy was one half hour twice a week. The therapist reinforced our private therapist's program.

The following year, Robin's high school schedule was language therapy, art, home economics, Future Farmers of America (FFA), chorus, and typing—no academics. Public school needed to be a positive experience. Robin was eighteen years old, and she graduated with a Certificate of Attendance.

Through all my home schooling and Robin's transition back into high school, she associated with typical people her own age. Even with all her issues, she felt equal to them because she too had worked really hard for her grades. Her peers didn't stay in high school until they were twenty-one, so why should she? Robin needed to move past high school.

Part III
Transitioning to Independent Adulthood

"Greatness is not in where we stand but in what direction we are moving. We must sail sometimes with the wind and sometimes against it—but sail we must and not drift, nor lie at anchor."

—Oliver Wendell Holmes

Chapter 8:
Employment

I was amazed at how much self-respect and self-confidence Robin gained when she got her first job. She was so proud of herself, and everyone in our community was proud of her. Despite the negative assumptions some professionals made about her employment prospects, she rose to the occasion. I put my fears and insecurities aside for her benefit. Bob and I set her up for success, and she succeeded. We just knew it was the right thing to do.

Employment is a normal developmental stage for everyone in life. Robin is no different. Many individuals with autism move from job to job because they haven't learned appropriate behaviors, responsibility, or basic employment skills. Even some experienced job coaches don't understand autism. It is important for parents to explore odd jobs, working during the summer, or working while attending school, if possible. Doesn't matter—just get a job with the benefit of a real paycheck.

On the other hand, state governments and businesses must encourage, support, and work toward including individuals with autism in the work force. It can be done by job carving, or customized employment, if necessary. Job carving is when a job description is modified to fit the individual. There are employment professionals who literally go into a work environment, identify skills their client *can* do to save other employee's time, and carve out a position just for their client. As examples:

- On the popular TV show "L.A. Law" (1986–1994), Benny, played by Larry Drake, was a character with obvious mental challenges. He was the *office boy*—running errands, making copies, getting coffee, and doing whatever else was requested of him. Benny was respected by his co-workers, and they cared about his personal life. (Benny helped fuel my vision for Robin's future.)
- A friend of Robin's got a job bagging groceries. She is good at bagging groceries but she cannot physically push the grocery cart to the customer's car in the parking lot. Another bagger steps in and takes her customer's groceries to their car.

Entering the Workforce

Robin has always wanted to work in an office; however, I was very protective of her self-image, and I knew she couldn't afford a long string of poor employment experiences. I had heard horror stories from other parents that concerned me. One example: A young adult who worked in a typing pool was isolated and verbally abused by her co-workers. The co-workers had no training to understand her disability and work with her, so it was easier for them to simply ignore her. Fortunately, this young lady became upset enough to tell her parents. They supported her and found her another job working with the public as a waitress. She was much happier.

I knew Robin's behaviors were much more appropriate in public than they were at home. She knew how to *perform*. However, I did not trust *typical* people to be nice to Robin, and I really didn't trust Robin to be nice to them when no one else was around.

In Robin's defense, her responses to people could be considered inappropriate. She didn't relate well to strangers, and her blank *stares* confused people. So just exactly, what did I want?

- I wanted Robin in a job where she was forced to relate to the public. I felt nothing could happen to her if people around her were watching.
- I wanted Robin in a job where she was accepted and given a chance. I didn't want to set her up for failure.
- I wanted Robin to be able to get back and forth to work independently.

Publix supermarket became the obvious choice to meet all my needs for Robin. A new store posted a *Now Hiring* sign near our home. It took Robin three days just to fill out the job application. I went with her for her interview. When they called Robin's name, I automatically stood up with her and the interviewer said to me, "You can stay here." *That's great,* I thought. They didn't get around the corner before the lady came back and said, "You can come too."

At the interview Robin was neat and clean. Her teeth were brushed and her hair was appropriate for a job interview. She was polite. She listened and did not monopolize the conversation; in fact, she hardly spoke. I felt the hiring manager saw potential in Robin as a valuable employee and wanted to help her succeed. All Robin was expected to do was to follow Publix handbook rules and do a good job.

Robin got the job and they trained her on how to use the time clock, where to find her hours each week, and how to bag groceries. For reinforcement, I went over the manual's rules with her, then pulled out my used grocery bags, emptied my kitchen cabinets, and she practiced bagging groceries.

Publix has front-end managers who monitor the baggers. Robin learned to ask them for help when she was confused. When necessary, they reminded her of her job responsibilities. Robin had regular written employment evaluations to keep her focused on areas where she needed to improve.

Many with autism, and their families, would rather not work than bag groceries. To these individuals I say, "Get over it." Any employment is power. No one should be denied that first paycheck. The first job is crucial to build other employment opportunities. Robin has learned important employment skills in her job at Publix:

- Making her job a priority in her life
- Learning good hygiene on the job
- Giving eye contact, smiling, saying, "Paper or plastic?" and acting appropriately
- Using traffic safety as she took customers' groceries to their cars
- Understanding responsibility and pride in Publix's rules and to do a good job
- Ignoring inappropriate behaviors of co-workers
- Getting to work on time and punching a time clock, including lunch
- Keeping track of her work schedule, which changes weekly
- Respecting her supervisors—she has to listen, follow instructions, and accept criticism gracefully
- Knowing where merchandise is in the store

Robin was able to meet all these goals, and she did not have a paid job coach. To support her employment, Bob also became a front-end bagger. This gave him a good relationship with the store managers and gave Robin the security blanket she needed for success. Bob worked only a couple of days a week, if that, and usually not on Robin's shift. The fact that he was an employee was just enough to keep Robin focused. We were careful not to overprotect her, and he slowly retired from his position.

Robin was a front-end bagger for six years. This responsibility gave her incredible relationships with the people in our community. She was very responsible, appropriate, and careful. Besides bagging groceries and helping customers to their cars, she had cart duty several times a day, returning carts from the parking lot back to their storage bin.

Promotions Can Happen

After Robin passed her driving learner's permit test, Nancy, the cashier trainer at Publix, asked me if Robin would like to be a cashier. She felt Robin should have the opportunity, since she had passed her driving test. I was flabbergasted. I talked with Robin, and she decided she wanted to try it. Robin loved the idea of wearing a cashier's uniform. Nancy called and asked me how to train Robin. I said, "Make sure you train her correctly the first time, because she doesn't retrain well."

I started a crash course to teach Robin money. She always had money in her pocket but couldn't understand the concept without being literal. For example, after church one Sunday, I asked Robin if I could borrow $10 to register for an event. Robin said, "I don't have $10." I was confused. Looking at her, I said, "Do you have $20?" She said, "Yes." I then borrowed $20 to pay for my $10 ticket.

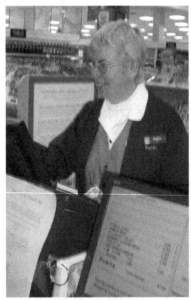

Fig. 8.1. Robin has been at Publix supermarket fifteen years.

One of Robin's first customers as a cashier was our neighbor Sandy. She went through Robin's line to buy groceries. The next day, Sandy went through Robin's line again. As Sandy was putting her items on the conveyor belt, she said to Robin, "I had to buy dog food today because I can't remember if I bought it yesterday." Robin said, "You bought six cans yesterday!"

Our community is very supportive of Robin. My phone rang for weeks with friends and neighbors calling to congratulate us on Robin's new position as cashier. She was beaming. Everyone was so proud of her as they went through her line at the store. Bob had long ago resigned as a *bagger*, but now he went back to work at Publix to support Robin. Our dinner table conversations revolved around how to solve problems as a cashier. It was like starting all over again for Robin. The following were some of the issues she struggled with:

- It was taking her too long to count her cash drawer.
- If a customer asked her a question while she was scanning their groceries, Robin would walk away without telling the customer she was going to get an answer. Needless to say, the customers were a little confused.
- Robin depended too much on the other cashiers. She was confused about some of the grocery items, because she didn't know where they were located in the store.
- She was insecure and lacked the confidence to speak up.

Robin is very proud of herself as a cashier. Mr. B., her store manager for over ten years, gave Robin the chance to succeed. Our family provided support by shopping there and having Bob work sporadically in the store. Publix is an incredible employer for individuals with developmental disabilities, including autism.

Expanding from Part-time to Full-time Work

The big question now became: *Can Robin work a forty-hour week?* We were concerned about Robin working at Publix full time standing in one position. We wanted to see if she could handle two part-time jobs.

Robin began volunteering at the Oldsmar City Clerk's Office. One of Robin's social group mothers was the city clerk. Robin worked in her office for over two years—filing, faxing, and mailing two half days a week. Robin loved the volunteering, and it was a wonderful opportunity for her. She learned she could handle a fuller schedule, and she liked working in an office. Robin likes politics, so becoming friends with the mayor was a special bonus!

Robin had a Social Security review during this time that included an updated psychological evaluation. Gerald J. Hodan, PhD, confirmed my concerns that I might be pushing Robin too hard and expecting too much. However, she was successful with volunteering and working at the same time.

Gerald J. Hodan, PhD, 2001 Social Security psychological evaluation

"Robin is basically a woman who is probably functioning at her highest level right now given she is doing so well as a cashier … she has learned to use the cash register very well to tell her exactly the amount of change to give someone."

We decided to experiment with two paying jobs. We requested a job coach through Robin's Home and Community Based Services (HCBS) Medicaid waiver for the next phase of her employment.

Robin's job coach helped Robin apply and interview for a membership receptionist position at our community YMCA. Robin got the job. This is a job that has been carved for Robin. She keeps the coffee bar full, greets customers, scans their membership card, and refers them to other receptionists for specific questions. She does not answer the phone.

The YMCA position was a different challenge for Robin, because of the social interactions they expect employees to have with their membership. She currently works ten hours a week, and she is working hard to improve her social skills as well as her office skills:

- Smiling at customers, making small talk, and saying their name as she checks them into the YMCA; wishing them "good morning" or "have a nice day," as appropriate
- Using the computer to identify members
- Looking busy and not gossiping
- Checking the coffee pots and keeping them full
- Making one-sided copies

Robin loves the variety that both jobs provide in her life. She started the YMCA position April 2007 and her Social Security has not been jeopardized, because she only does a percentage of the receptionist job description. She seriously thought about quitting when her shift changed to 7:00 a.m. I explained to her that in the *real world,* everybody has parts of their job they would rather change. She gets up at 5:30 a.m. to be at work before 7:00 a.m. It could be worse—her supervisor starts work at 4 a.m.

The Importance and Attainability of Employment

Never assume that your young adult cannot be successfully employed. As a parent, it is easy to overprotect and smother our children with love, when in fact we need to be planning their future. The school system protects school-age students, then passes that responsibility back to the parents when they are done. But are parents ready?

It is important parents help their child with autism reach for the *brass ring*, employment. Most states provide assistance, if necessary, and I have seen some incredible stories of success. Parents need to celebrate employment, because many support services and opportunities revolve around the *haves* and the *have-nots*.

- Those that have employment in their life receive positive support to be independent and a part of their community (example: language therapy in adulthood).
- Those that have no employment in their life are not encouraged to grow and develop into the person they might be.

Robin's employment opportunity at Publix gave her the self-image I could never provide at home. She learned, like other adults, that the world is not about her, and she has been able to build on that confidence in other areas of her life. I've been asked many times, "How did you do it? Aren't you afraid for her?" Of course I am, but I also realized, as Robin's mother, that I had to *let go and let God!* Bob and I have developed a safety net to the best of our ability, and that's the best we can do.

Chapter 9:
Community Inclusion—Self-Determination

"In our search to achieve social justice for people with disabilities, we have determined that there are fundamental flaws in the manner in which this nation has created a system of 'community' services that frequently fosters isolation from community. We are painfully aware, that, though well intended, this separation causes people to be perceived as 'different.' Their quality of life suffers. Their basic human rights may be jeopardized. How, we asked over and over again, can we change this?"

—Tom Nerney, Center for Self-Determination[18]

Thankfully, people like Tom Nerney were thinking about self-determination and true inclusion in the community long before I realized it was my priority. Admittedly, I was not prepared for Robin's adulthood. I assumed Robin would always be a part of *our* lives—not have her own life and her own friends.

Patty, a friend, convinced me to attend a self-determination conference held in Atlanta, Georgia, over ten years ago. By this time, Robin was already working. We felt very content and successful with the progress we'd made with her, and I was reluctant to go to the conference. But go I did, and it was there I learned that individuals with disabilities deserve respect and independence, not structure and boundaries. I learned the importance of individual freedom rather than being victims of poverty and abuse. I clearly began to understand the phrase *nothing about me without me*. I realized:

- I was still treating Robin like a child.
- I let my fear of the dangers in today's society smother her life.
- I didn't trust Robin, or anybody else, taking my job as her protector.
- I didn't show Robin the same trust and respect I showed her sisters and other adults.
- I was going to have to change my way of *looking* at Robin if I expected anyone else to do the same.

---

18 www.self-determination.com.

Many individuals with autism exhibit inappropriate behaviors because they're frustrated and angry. Although Robin and I have a good relationship, she often took her anger out on me. Besides anger, she was easily overwhelmed and anxious. I, on the other hand, was battling my own fears that other people wouldn't understand her. I honestly thought she wasn't ready for any kind of independence. Therefore, my excuse was always, *she's not ready yet*. Patty always reminded me, "You're never ready if you have a developmental disability—just do it." I unexpectedly grew that weekend. I saw things I approved of and things I definitely did not approve of, but I grew. I grew for the benefit of Robin.

People with developmental disabilities, including autism, were originally *out of the community*, meaning they were in institutions or homebound from society and the school system. In the 1970s, Public Law 94-142: *Education of All Handicapped Children Act* became law. Now known as the *Individual with Disabilities Education Act (IDEA)*, it started the standard of moving individuals with disabilities *into* the community—for an education. For individuals with autism, moving *into* the community just isn't good enough. Today, we must embrace the self-determination movement, which supports making individuals *a part* of the community, including the possibility of employment and supported or independent living.

As Robin entered the adult world, she still depended on me, and I knew I had the power to make her a part of her community. Receiving my education from the self-determination movement, my focus became my personal definition of self-determination. I admired their goals, but for Robin, I knew what she could handle best because of her autism.

It was a very confusing time for me. Just what did I want for her? We moved to Florida thinking we had *a plan* for Robin, only to see our own motives and direction challenged. The more I got involved in the adult disability community, the more opportunities I saw for her future. I worked hard to keep an open mind, and I slowly moved forward seeking her unknown future. She couldn't do this alone.

Understanding the Dynamics of Independence with Autism

Some people with autism literally define independence to mean "I'll do it myself. I don't need you anymore!" Are any of us truly independent? I'm married. I'm definitely not independent. People need people. That's what makes us all human. Yet people with autism can easily end up in unnecessary isolation that removes them from family and friends—because of their literal interpretation of independence.

I met a gentleman, John, living in an assisted living facility (ALF). John's mother had died and his father was in a nursing home. John's sister wanted to continue being a part of her brother's life but she had no legal recourse to make it happen. She did not have guardianship. The ALF administration followed and taught, to the letter, their definition of independence and they interpreted true independence to include separation from family and previous friendships. John supported and agreed with the ALF's definition to the extreme of isolating himself from his sister, like a rebellious teenager.

Without the help of the ALF to support healthy family relationships, John does not see his sister. She has no legal avenue to reestablish contact, and policies have made him a ward of the state without any freedom or choice. This situation is very sad.

Considering Guardianship and Durable Power of Attorney

When Robin was eighteen years old, I filed for and received full guardianship over her, meaning I now had total control. I feared professionals would treat her as a client or customer rather than a person. I'd heard horror stories from other families and actually met some of those very social workers over the years. There was no way this was going to happen to my daughter. I knew her needs best, and I thought guardianship was my answer. I'd worked too long and too hard to lose control as she reached adulthood. Perhaps you can see the problem here: I had made it all about me!

Robin was embarrassed every time something needed a signature, because others always wanted my signature, not hers. She couldn't have a checking account, she couldn't vote, she couldn't sign her condominium contract, she couldn't have a credit card, and she couldn't drive. Guardianship was limiting her opportunities to be an independent adult. She deserved better.

Ten years after working so hard to get full guardianship of Robin, I had all her rights restored, meaning my guardianship was removed. It's much easier to take a person's rights away than to restore them. I made a drastic, unnecessary, and expensive error in judgment trying to protect my child. It was expensive, and even then, I now realize full guardianship was not necessary.

I found an attorney who agreed to help me restore Robin's legal rights to allow her to make her own decisions. We went to court, and I testified in a chair next to the judge's bench, like you see on TV. The judge asked me several questions and then instructed me to step down. The judge then looked at Robin, who sat at a table with her attorney, and asked her if she had anything to add. Without hesitation, Robin immediately began correcting my testimony. I was so proud. Everyone in the room quietly chuckled! The judge looked at my attorney smiling and said, "Her rights are restored." Today, Bob, Robin, and I have durable power of attorney on each other. Durable power of attorney on Robin transfers to her sisters upon our death.

I am Robin's Social Security representative payee, ensuring that the bookkeeping meets their guidelines. Currently, a Social Security representative payee does not need guardianship to be responsible for an individual's Social Security benefits.

In most states, before a young adult reaches eighteen years old, a parent needs to decide what they are going to do about guardianship. Some families do find it necessary to have guardianship for medical and financial purposes only, but alternatives should be considered before automatically jumping into full or limited guardianship decisions.

- Ask your child's primary care doctor about *health care surrogate* or *health care proxy*, whatever is available in your state. Setting this up in advance can be very important for medical interventions. A procedure as simple as a wisdom tooth extraction can easily become a maze of emergency legal paperwork in the court system. Will your young adult give permission, if necessary?
- A popular alternative to guardianship for some families is a *microboard*. This is an excellent way to bring parents, siblings, and community members working together for the benefit of a person with autism. The nonprofit organization's sole purpose is the care of one specific individual. A microboard helps to establish community support for an individual and relieves siblings of sole responsibility after their parents' deaths. The Tennessee Microboards Association is committed to the development of high quality comprehensive services and supports to children and adults with disabilities in a manner that fosters self-determination and inclusion. They have many success stories and are available for help and guidance.[19]

---

19 www.microboards.org.

Do be aware: if you need to continue being a part of your child's educational decisions after eighteen years of age, you may need to send legal documentation to the school system to allow your participation in educational decisions. Parents may be denied access to school information and meetings about their child because the school system considers the child an adult at eighteen years of age.

Every state has different options for guardianship. This has been an expensive lesson for our family. Listen to other parents. An attorney who specializes in this field may be able to help you make the right choices. Special needs trusts, living wills, health care surrogate, health care proxy, and durable power of attorney are terms you need to be familiar with as your child becomes an adult.

A simple example: Robin kept complaining about a bruise on the top of her thigh. I thought she had bruised it in karate class. She said it didn't hurt. She repeatedly complained about it for several months and I realized it wasn't going away. I watched as it slowly developed into a hard, purplish dried pea-shaped knot.

Robin's chiropractor and local MD both said it was probably a wooden splinter and it would eventually dissolve on its own. Still concerned, I asked a surgeon friend to look at it. He did a biopsy. Diagnosis: It was an extremely rare cancerous tumor: *Dermatofibrosarcoma protuberans*.

Robin agreed to the surgery and we did not need to use our durable power of attorney. She has an indented six-inch scar on her leg today. The cancer had not gone through to the muscle or bone, and there have been no reoccurrences to date.

The Importance of Respect

People's lives are so busy today we forget that our *words* matter. The general population, including myself, must learn to be more respectful of individuals with disabilities. Parents can no longer say, "My child's autistic." They should say, "My child has autism." This may sound like mere semantics to some, but to the individual with autism, it can be the difference between tearing down self-image and building up self-image, self-respect, and self-determination.

The word "autistic" is just one example. I have autism. I'm a person first who just happens to also have autism. I can be described in many ways other than in terms of my disability. I have a red jacket, I have blonde hair, I have autism. Robin's life is important to her, and it's important for people around her to respect this.

Parents must be the leaders, using the correct terms and appropriate language to refer to autistic people, or better said, *people with autism*. If we as parents want to promote inclusion, transition, and self-determination for our child or adult, we must set the tone. To be a part of the community, teachers, professionals, providers, media representatives, and even other family members need to be using respectful terms. Then, just maybe, respect will begin to affect change.

Cultivating Opportunities for Conscious Choice-making

My biggest fear was not Robin's independence. My biggest fear was the definition of choice and other people smothering Robin's independence by forcing their choices on her. Robin definitely has her own opinions and ideas. She isn't a follower, but she has followed most of her life because of her limited communication skills. When asked a question, Robin would stare at the person and they assumed her answer. That's not choice. People around Robin needed to understand her language disability and give her legitimate choices and the time to process the information so she could try and answer their questions. For example:

WRONG: Do you want to go to the mall?

CORRECT: Do you want to go to the mall *or* go to the pool? If you get no response, or a stare, give another set of choices.

Many parents, friends, and caretakers use the excuse "It was her choice" to justify something *they* want, not what the person with autism wants. Making an incorrect statement like this caused Robin to become anxious and frustrated. She knew it was not her choice but that she couldn't always express herself properly. Here are some examples of the ways the person with autism can have their responses misinterpreted:

- "She wanted to go to the mall." (Robin didn't want to go to the mall. The companion needed to check out a sale.)
- "He wanted hotdogs for dinner." (He'd had hotdogs every night for dinner for six weeks.)
- "He likes staying up late at night and watching TV." (No one explained to him that he can't keep a job because he's always tired from lack of sleep.)
- "She doesn't want to work." (No one is encouraging employment.)

Support providers, professionals, caretakers, community, and, yes, parents confuse *choice* with *choose*. You cannot *choose* something if you do not know or understand the options and consequences of the choices you make. Choice cannot be legislated. For some individuals, portions of their brain do not allow them to make stable choices or learn from consequences. These individuals need to fall back on the values of their family life for their boundaries. It's sad when a good support system is not in place and the consequences are illicit drugs, prostitution, crime, prison, and/or mental health confinement.

For individuals with classic autism, *choice* may need to be explained at their level of understanding—every single time. Even then, health and safety must be explained and play an important role in the final outcome of *choice*. We have spent years teaching Robin assertiveness and responsibility, and it has paid off!

Chapter 10:
Moving Out: Independent Living

"Thank God for cell phones."

Robin had already been working for several years when she began receiving state provider services through the Medicaid waiver at twenty-eight years old. Robin's waiver coordinator kept asking, "When are you going to start working on Robin's goals for independent living?" I thought I was. Robin had a job. She had a life with her friends in her social group, Mainstreamed Adult Singles at Home (MASH). She was driving, and she had a car, which gave her independence. She was singing in her church choir. Why rock the boat? She was fine. I didn't think having her own home was necessary or a reality. My attitude was, let them both dream. I knew I had the final say. Where was the money coming from? With Robin's income, she couldn't afford an apartment, and she definitely couldn't handle a roommate. She was her own best friend.

Independent living for Robin would be impossible without our moral support. To me, several factors determined whether she could live independently.

- Although Robin was receiving three hours of language therapy a week, her communication and language skills were still very poor.
- Robin did not understand the importance of a friendship. Therefore, she had no friends or anyone she wanted to room with.
- Robin still needed us for her survival.

I kept telling myself, she's not ready yet to live on her own. I finally shared my concerns with the coordinator. The bottom line was that we couldn't afford for Robin to live independently from us. This wasn't in our *plan* when we retired. We couldn't supplement Robin's income. In addition, I knew Robin's life was successful only because we controlled her boundaries with structure and consistency.

The coordinator gave me two phone numbers to call for housing information. I felt compelled to follow through. God was obviously on Robin's side. It was November. The local housing authority said they had two low-income housing loans available. They were first come, first serve and expired in two months. The mortgage had to be in Robin's name. Even though she was still receiving Social Security Disability Income (SSDI), she qualified because:

- She had a good employment record.
- She had no debt.
- She could make a down payment of $500.

Robin qualified for a $57,000 loan. Bob and I had a long talk with her and she really wanted to be more independent and live separate from us. She liked the idea of having her own home.

Robin was definitely progressing beyond our vision, and we thought she deserved this opportunity. Her resurgence of weekly language therapy at twenty-eight years old, along with her new gluten-free casein-free (GFCF) diet, along with vitamins and supplements, was bringing her to another whole level of capabilities (see chapter 2: Diet, Vitamins, and Supplements— and chapter 4: Speech and Language Therapy). Bob and I knew we were holding her back.

I went to work collecting paperwork for Robin's mortgage qualifications. A MASH member had just purchased a condominium within two miles of our house. I called his mom, because I knew she had recently researched affordable housing in our area. We liked the neighborhood where her son lived. Robin could qualify for a one-bedroom condominium. That decision was easy! A friend, Jack, had just completed his real estate license the week before. Jack wrote a letter to all thirteen homeowners of one-bedroom condominiums, telling them he had a buyer. The next day, Jack was playing golf with Bob when his cell phone rang. The lady on the other end of the line said, "Do you really have a buyer?" Jack said yes, and Robin signed the contract that afternoon.

At Thanksgiving, Heather, Robin's cousin, gave her a six-week-old kitten as a roommate. Robin hadn't done well with house pets in the past, and a pet never entered my mind. This was incredible—it gave Robin and Snowball several months together before the big move. She now had a roommate.

Hiring a Supported Living Coach

Finding a good support person is critical for the successful independence of a person with autism. Robin and I interviewed and hired a supported living coach through the HCBS waiver. Robin was so excited to move. Ginger, my sister, gave Robin a housewarming shower, and all our church friends showered Robin with gifts for her condominium. We gave Robin half the furniture we had, and we helped her move in, cat and all.

The state supported living coach we hired was a disaster and lasted less than one month. She didn't understand autism. She was distorting the truth and making excuses, which really upset Robin. Frustrated and confused, Robin was calling me more than twenty times a day. I couldn't put the fires out fast enough. The coach expected Robin to follow instructions between visits. She was spending Robin's startup funds on expensive foods and ignoring budget restrictions. In addition, Robin was upset with the coach because of her personal cell phone calls from family and friends. Obviously, Robin and I needed to develop better interview skills and instincts to help her find the right support person.

I was so ready for providers to take the lead with Robin. Robin, however, was not ready. I was so thankful we only lived two miles away. We were in emergency mode! We didn't have time to interview another state provider and gamble on another failure. Robin just wanted to be left alone, she didn't understand. She was once again foot stomping in frustration and slamming doors to communicate. Her behaviors were way off any chart, and I was afraid I'd made a terrible mistake.

On top of all this confusion for Robin, I realized she had to be taught the simplest of life's rules. As an example, we had a circle of support meeting at Robin's condo shortly after her move. I felt everyone needed to come together to support and evaluate her shaky transition. As conversation, I casually asked Robin what she did in the evenings, assuming it was watching TV. She said, "I go to the 7-11." I asked what time, and she said, "11 p.m."

There was dead silence in the room. After I calmed myself down, I explained the danger of any woman going out at 11 p.m. alone. This was one of the many lessons I realized I'd never *taught* Robin. Throughout her childhood, Bob always made a night-store run for the next morning's bread or milk. She didn't see the difference until I explained it to her.

We needed to start over with a more positive transition plan for Robin, and fortunately, the HCBS waiver coordinator agreed with me. I turned to a dear friend, Elaine, who quickly stepped in to rescue Robin as her supported living coach. Elaine had patience with Robin and genuinely cared about her. She became her friend and her provider. Elaine respected Robin, and Robin knew it. She gave Robin the space and time she needed to understand her newfound independence and learn how to make good choices. Elaine was Robin's *life preserver* for the next two years.

Just adding another person to Robin's life was overwhelming for her. She was so fragile in those early days, and we all learned to tiptoe around her mood swings. When Elaine and I sit and talk about those early days, it's amazing how Robin has changed. It's also amazing Elaine stuck with us. It wasn't easy.

Robin no longer acts out her frustrations and she is much more in control of her life. To help Robin understand, I developed a chart to show the importance of being responsible and assertive for oneself. Robin needed to realize she didn't want a substitute mother to manage her. She needed to do it herself.

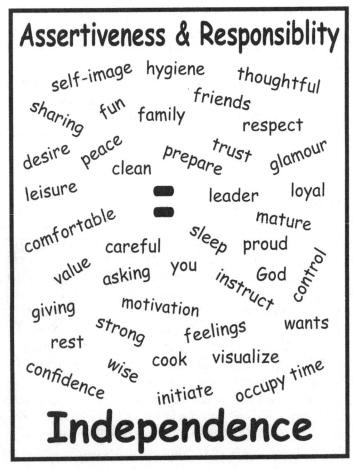

Fig. 14.1. Assertiveness and Responsibility Chart.

Michelle has been Robin's supported living coach for over five years now. She lives three miles from Robin and is a supported living coach through the HCBS waiver. Michelle and Robin are the same age, truly like each other, and have fun. Michelle is honest and a good role model. She doesn't lie or exaggerate, which is critical for Robin. They share a lot of personal experiences, which has really helped Robin value the people around her.

Michelle and I keep in touch. We had a meeting at Robin's condominium, and I didn't realize Michelle's St. Bernard dog, BJ, had been very sick. While we were all busily greeting each other at the doorway, Robin interrupted, and she asked Michelle, "How is BJ?" Michelle burst out crying. Robin stretched her arms equally around Michelle's neck and comforted her until Michelle regained her composure. Michelle had just come from burying BJ. Michelle and I locked eyes, and we were amazed at Robin's appropriateness and compassion. Michelle pulled out her cell phone and showed Robin pictures of BJ, just before he died and her family burying him in their backyard. She shared with Robin the details of BJ's last hours alive. Throughout all this, Robin totally focused on Michelle and her needs, showing genuine compassion.

Michelle recently helped Robin give a Christmas Open House for her condominium neighbors. Elaine and her husband, Bill, were invited. Elaine commented to me what a true friendship they have and how well Robin and Michelle work together. Their friendship is very obvious to the people they meet.

Managing Autism-driven Compulsiveness

I feel Robin's compulsiveness is as much my fault as it is her fault. (Admittedly, we were never consistent with allowances.) Living with us, she always followed the family rules and we approved her purchases. She knew what I would approve! Living alone, Robin now had the freedom to spend her own money. This spending problem never entered my mind—until crisis spending presented itself. Thus, I have taken the challenge to help her develop responsible money management.

Before Robin moved into her condominium, on the recommendation of a provider, I put Robin on the prescription drug Prozac from her local doctor. I knew Robin's transition to independent living was going to be difficult, never imagining how difficult. After Robin's move, she continued her vitamins, supplements, and the Prozac but stopped the GFCF diet—I thought the diet was too difficult for her to manage. We saw no benefit from the Prozac. Within six months, Robin gained over forty pounds—130 to 174 pounds.

Desperate, I called Dr. Bradstreet, Robin's autism doctor, and he helped us wean Robin off the Prozac.

Robin was gaining two-and-a-half pounds a week, and I thought she had developed some sort of disease. I knew I was not the person to implement weight management so I took her to a recommended chiropractor. He saw her weekly for two years, with adjustments, weigh-ins, and pep talks. He said that although her hands weren't flapping (stimming), she was having severe internal stimming behaviors. His weekly adjustments seemed to help her anxiety. I tried to remove myself from this situation and let him take the lead.

Well, there was no disease! It took me two years to finally realize that Robin was buying $10 worth of candy, sodas, and cookies daily. She was on a chemical high. The chiropractor tried telling me this, but I wouldn't listen. Oh, no, not my daughter! Robin was lying about everything to the chiropractor, Bob, and me! Lying was a new developmental skill for her. I couldn't believe it.

Controlling Compulsive Eating

Honesty is important to diet. Desperate, I became the gatekeeper of Robin's debit card, money, and checkbook. When I called Dr. Bradstreet, he confirmed compulsiveness can be a serious issue for people with autism. Robin's primary disability now was binge eating. She was obsessed with food. Her weight was a battle I seriously thought was not important on the scale of things, but a weight gain of two-and-a-half pounds a week had to stop. She looked like a balloon that was about to pop. Regrouping, and on the advice of Robin's local doctor, I was determined I was not going to lose this weight battle!

I talked with Robin. She must have emotional *buy-in* to solve her weight problem. It was affecting her self-image. We discussed options, and she decided to sign up for the Jenny Craig diet program. It's a bargain compared to what she was spending, and it gave her the structure and boundaries she needed.

Taking a week's supply of Jenny Craig food home didn't work for Robin either. She was eating everything in two days. Now it was time to regroup again. The food came to my house, and she'd stopped by after work each day to pick up the next day's food supply. That worked! The following year, she took all the food to her house—except snacks and desserts. Those were still too tempting!

When Robin saw Dr. Bradstreet for her annual visit, he was very impressed with her weight loss and excited for her. I shared my concerns with him that

Robin still needed someone controlling her boundaries, and although she appeared appropriate, she was anxious and angry at times, which limited her independence. He did a blood test for yeast, and it was negative. He recommended that Robin go back on the GFCF diet. (Duh, I never thought of that!)

Compulsive Purchases

Robin can be very compulsive in her purchases, too. During this same period with food, she obsessed over anything with the Tampa Bay Buccaneers (Bucs) football insignia on it. She had three heavy quilted winter Bucs coats in her closet, and we live in Florida. Trying to stay positive, I asked her why she bought the XL man's coat, and she answered, "They didn't have it in medium." All coats were different, yet all had the Bucs insignia on them. We joked about it, saying that she didn't need three heavy coats, and I thought we'd agreed on restricting the purchase of *all* Bucs products unless they won the Super Bowl again. I thought that was a reasonable compromise. As we watched football games and saw products in the stores, I would comment on how nice they were—but not to purchase.

Robin was going on a job interview and needed a new blouse. I suggested she and Michelle go shopping, with a $25 limit. They came home with a $70 Bucs shirt for her job interview! Michelle knew better, but state administrators feel individuals should learn from their mistakes. Under normal circumstances, I might agree, but Robin's compulsive issues from her autism require guidance to help her learn appropriate choices, consequences, and decisions.

Learning to Budget and Spend Wisely

Michelle is excellent at helping Robin with her household responsibilities. However, I felt she was too close to Robin to help her recognize her compulsiveness and budget her money. Robin and I decided she needed a separate supported living coach to help with budget and finances. I stepped back and let him take over. The goal was for him to help Robin live within a budget and spend her money responsibly.

Robin was confident writing her checks and balancing her monthly bank statements, using Quicken. This had been her structure for several years. This new supported living coach was trying to set Robin's computer up so it would automatically download bank transactions into Quicken. Robin was upset because she couldn't understand her money anymore. After several weeks, things were getting no better so I politely suggested he was confusing her. I reminded him his goal was to help her learn to *budget*. He taught Robin how to do her own credit check, and they decided to apply for a VISA card. I knew how this was going to turn out, but I said nothing. Two months later, Robin brought me her VISA bill, with $340 worth of things she now had to pay for. I asked for the statement receipts, which she gladly provided. I was very disappointed this new coach didn't recognize his responsibility to help Robin monitor her credit card spending, much less implement *budgeting*.

For Robin's survival, I helped her get her finances back in order, and we currently work on this together, when necessary. Finances are the most critical area that can limit Robin's true independence. However, I learned I cannot expect someone else to teach her budgeting when I had failed. I needed to do it myself!

Building a Reliable Support Staff

I realize the day will come when we can no longer be in Robin's life. We're definitely replaceable; however, my biggest concern is the learning curve of her new providers. This close and personal interaction with an inappropriate person could easily encourage her autism behaviors to reappear.

Trying to meet this need, a friend suggested I purchase the book, *All Cats Have Asperger Syndrome*, by Kathy Hoopman (Jessica Kingsley Publishers, 2006). This book gave me the vision to write one just for Robin, *Ode to My Staff*. Each page has a picture of Robin, emphasizing a particular uniqueness or concern she has. Sample pages include:

- Respect me. Don't talk *about* me, talk *to* me. Remember— *nothing about me without me.*
- I expect you to be totally honest with me—at all times.
- Please make sure I'm eating a gluten-free casein-free diet, sleeping well, and taking my vitamins properly.
- Do not enable me. I can do it myself, but I may not realize I need your support to make that happen.
- Have patience with me, and give me time to complete a task. In other words, don't rush me.
- I do need change in my life. Push me to try new things even though I say no. I can get my priorities mixed up sometimes and I think my routine is more important than trying something new.
- Don't allow me to get stuck by my *autism force*.

- Sometimes I get frustrated, but it's not because of things you think I'm frustrated about. My brain gets overloaded and all mixed up sometimes and I can't clearly tell you why I'm anxious or upset.
    - Example: I appear angry when you call. Actually, I'm angry because you didn't call me last night, as you said you would, and I don't want to talk to you today.
- I don't see obvious things other people see, yet these are important to me. Someone needs to keep me on track.
    - Example: I need you to help me review my closet and remind me when to purchase new clothes.
- I need you to remind me of health and safety issues because I forget the importance of safety rules and recognizing danger.
    - Example: Sometimes I come home after dark, and I forget to check my surroundings when getting out of my car. Also, I forget and carry too many bags into the house when I can get them in the morning, when it's light outside.
- Remember, I need love and encouragement, an occasional bit of advice, and a hug once in a while.

Handling Frustrating Events

I went with Robin to language therapy because I needed to talk with the therapist. The parking lot cars were tightly spaced. As Robin carefully opened her door, she tapped the car door next to us. The woman in the other car went into a screaming rage at Robin. Robin scrambled out of the car and stood in the middle of the parking lot, confused and doing her autism dance. (Robin's *autism dance* consists of full body movements, often in a circular motion.) The woman got out of her car and continued screaming at Robin. I got out of the car and calmly told Robin to go into the therapy center. I would handle it.

Not being able to calm the woman down, I finally said, in a firm voice, "Listen, she has *autism*, and you have parked in an *autism* zone." As I said this, I pointed to the therapy center sign. The woman immediately calmed down, got back in her car, and I went inside and confirmed to Robin she'd done nothing wrong. Actually, I was a little afraid of the woman myself.

Somehow, the word "autism" gave the woman a sense of perspective. I told Robin she really needs to be able to use the word autism to control or stabilize situations in an emergency. This was an emergency, and the "autism dance" needs modification. Robin now carries a card in her wallet about autism, to show others if needed.

Balancing Work and Play

Robin's cell phone has given her the independence she wanted. This is her lifeline. Many times she has called and said, "I need Dad, now." This usually involves car problems. If she has any questions or concerns, she doesn't hesitate to call. We've learned not to panic. Robin is very assertive and responsible for what Robin wants to be assertive and responsible for, which is a lot.

- She is a very responsible driver. She never goes over the speed limit and makes sure her car is well maintained and clean.
- She is very responsible towards Snowball and loves her dearly.
- Her laundry and housekeeping are always up to date.
- She independently pays her bills on time, and she's never late for work.

Keeping busy is important for Robin's motivational needs. She does that best, whether working, going for a walk, swimming at her community pool, working out at the YMCA, attending MASH social activities, visiting us, or shopping. She has no time for anxiousness, depression or loneliness.

Robin needs to learn to relax and enjoy her life. This can be difficult for a person with autism, and she does not recognize this as a problem. Thus, we added a HCBS waiver companion to her schedule. Carolyn comes to Robin's house on Tuesdays in the late afternoon. The goal is for Robin to enjoy cooking for Carolyn and just hanging out in her own place. They do their fingernails together, play games, cook (GFCF), take power walks around Robin's complex, and watch TV. (I think Robin channel surfs when home alone). Carolyn says Robin is cooking a balanced meal, and she enjoys having company for dinner. This growth has resulted in Robin having friends over for dinner, games, and movie night.

Robin's Life Today

Robin has been in her condominium for eight years now. All of these traumatic moments are behind her. She's still on the GFCF diet, but she can now successfully cheat on occasion. She no longer calls us to ask where to set her thermostat or what clothes to wear. Her kitchen cabinets are full of

GFCF food, and she is responsible for her grocery shopping. Her money and credit cards are still in my purse in her blue billfold. She independently gets her cards, does what she needs, and puts them back on her next visit. I never question her bills. She now pays them directly through her bank's Web site. She sees no need to carry cash!

Robin is not afraid to ask for help and we willingly support her. Yes, we are definitely her *staff*. She takes the lead in keeping us, and herself, organized. She is the *queen* of lists and charts! Periodically, I ask her if she wants a roommate, and the answer is always no.

Robin is very comfortable with her independent life. She has a lot of confidence. People in our community see her as a cheerful and successful independent woman. Her success is due to the quality supports she's had—state providers and community—working with her family.

As Robin's parents, we gave her the space and time she has needed for learning her independence, and we recognized the necessary steps to reach each goal.

Part IV
Our Family Supporting Robin

"Expect more than others think is possible;
Dream more than others think is practical;
Risk more than others think is safe."

—Benjamin Franklin

Chapter 11:
Our Experience as Parents

Never take for granted the importance of a good marriage when you have a child with autism. Bob and I have always respected each other and have always gotten along (well, almost always). We are best friends. He is an easygoing person, thank God, and it takes a lot to get him angry—then, watch out! If I believed in luck, I'd say I'm very lucky!

I was a secretary and Bob was a flight-line mechanic for the Air National Guard when we married. After our marriage, we saved to purchase our first home and started our family. Life was much simpler forty years ago. Our biggest decisions were purchasing a house, a car, and a vacation. He traveled a lot with his new job and I was a stay-at-home mom. In those days, fathers brought home the weekly paycheck and had *fun* with their children. Mothers managed the home, including the children. I was the family bookkeeper, and Bob always agreed with my financial decisions as long as I stayed within budget.

Bob and I had been married for ten years when Robin was born. Pam was seven and Karen was five years old. We were a typical family with two young girls.

While I was pregnant with Robin, Bob and I decided we needed a larger house with another bedroom for Robin. We purchased a new home and visited the construction site most weekends. After Robin was born, we continued these weekend trips and moved when she was three months old. These trips became a good diversion while Robin "recovered" from her medical doctor's diagnosis of colic. As parents of a third child, we knew something was very wrong with Robin and knew that her continual screaming had nothing to do with colic. On this drive we passed an old two-room schoolhouse with a sign that read, "Muriel Humphrey School for Retarded Children" before reaching our new home. I would tear up every time we passed it and wonder, "Will Robin go to this school?"

Bob and I were Sunday school teachers for the senior high class at church. They loved going through the stages of my pregnancy with me. These girls babysat, and they knew something was very wrong with Robin. The haunting looks on their faces confirmed our fears. They wanted to hold

Robin but couldn't. The weekly church newsletter even had a cartoon of us holding Robin in her awkward face-down position, printed as a joke. Nobody knew what to say to us.

I took Robin to JC Penney at two-and-a-half months old to have a professional baby picture taken. We had pictures of the other girls at that age, and I wanted one of Robin as well. The young photographer taking Robin's picture looked at me and said, "You know, there's something wrong with her." The photographer couldn't get Robin to hold her head up or stop screaming for the picture.

"Yes, I know," I said.

A friend called after a Sunday baptism of another child and asked, "Are you and Bob getting a divorce?" She sat in the choir loft and saw I was crying as I watched the baptism of another baby.

"No," I said. "I wish it were that simple." I shared our fears with her about Robin.

Our life, like those of many other families with autism, was turning upside down. We knew nothing about the world of disability—nothing. That's something that happened to other people, not us.

When Robin was a year old, one of her doctors in the Birth Defects Clinic, Children's Hospital National Medical Center, Washington, D.C., recommended that we place Robin in an institution for the benefit of our other children. Seeing the blank expression on my face and my lack of response, he then said, "As long as she's progressing, be thankful."

Funny, how this comment has stayed with me—"as long as she's progressing." This was the vision we needed. I clearly remember praying, "Lord, I can do this if you are with me." Sure enough, he has never left my side. He is still with me, and Robin is still progressing!

Making Marriage a Continual Partnership

As Robin's disabilities became more apparent, loneliness became a major factor in our lives. Just surviving each day was our reality. Many friends withdrew and relatives didn't understand because, admittedly, it was all I talked about. I felt guilty that I couldn't make Robin better. I was exhausted and short tempered. My mood swings often paralleled Robin's behavior.

If it wasn't for Robin's continual screaming, I think we would have accepted her slow development. We both honestly felt she was in pain, crying out to us for help. Our first big decision was simple: find out what was wrong with Robin, regardless of the cost. Why is she screaming? She wasn't like this her first month of life. We were desperate for answers. I made appointment after appointment with medical professions seeking answers. When they couldn't help her, we were both so discouraged.

Bob was always supportive and understanding, and we never doubted each other or blamed each other for our circumstances.

Memories are so personal. The longing for eye contact, affection or hugs, the advice from friends on how to raise our child and their assurances we just needed to discipline her more, the frustration of sitting in doctors' offices expecting some type of pill or answer. We quickly learned that our family was on our own.

Determined to help Robin, I took the lead for our family, but I didn't make any decisions without Bob's full support. I needed to respect his judgments and he needed to respect mine. To do this, we both had to educate ourselves—not him depending on my judgments and decisions.

I headed to the public library to do my research. There wasn't much there in 1971, and everything was too technical for me anyway. I didn't understand the medical language when it came to disability. I did find a book about Montessori school teachings that opened our eyes and I realized 'inappropriate behavior is unacceptable in society.' This realization scared us. What kind of future would Robin have?

I searched magazine articles, gave them to Bob, and said, "Read this." In the 1970s, *Woman's Day* magazine had an article almost every month on disabilities or child development. We both read them all. These articles gave us opportunities for discussion and reminded us that things could be worse. When appropriate, we shared them with doctors. While professionals never appreciated the facts that we related from *Woman's Day* magazine, these short, concise articles gave us the variety of knowledge we needed, and they opened our eyes to choices and possibilities. Other magazine articles and books were surfacing about disabilities at the same time:

- In 1975 a pediatric allergist from California proposed that artificial colors and flavors, preservatives, and salicylates caused hyperactivity in children. Benjamin Feingold, MD, wrote *Why Your Child Is Hyperactive* (Random House, 1975-1985). It was the first book I had heard about that linked behaviors to food.
- The Philadelphia Institute for the Achievement of Human Potential taught a rigid one-to-one program concentrating on helping children with physical disabilities. The system of *patterning* was devised by physical therapist Glenn J. Doman and psychologist Carl Delacato. It required intense structure for

a child during waking hours, including help from community volunteers. Doman[20] and Delacato[21] are still involved in child development today.

- As an occupational therapist, A. Jean Ayres, PhD, studied brain development in the 1970s. Dr. Ayres's book, *Sensory Integration and the Child* (Western Psychological Services, 1979-2005) established the importance of the body's development as it relates directly to the brain. She realized some people could not process information, including behaviors and tasks, the same way that others did. A new specialty field of occupational therapy sensory integration (OT/SI) was based on Dr. Ayers's research.

- *Son Rise: A Miracle of Love,* by Barry Kauffman (Harbor & Row, 1976) was published and was made into a television movie. It was about the recovery of his child with autism. I felt the Kauffman family was *patterning* similar to the Philadelphia Institute.

None of these breakthroughs in the 1970s were supported by the mainstream medical community—none. As we skipped from MD to MD, their recommendations were always the same: "There's nothing we can do" or "Let's wait and see." They focused more on me, *the mother,* as the real problem, because I didn't accept Robin as she was. I wanted to change her, fix her. Bob and I quietly listened. How could we defend ourselves? We ignored them, moving on to find help elsewhere.

Bob and I were raised with the belief that doctors were next to God and could do no harm. They were the epitome of knowledge. As we became disillusioned by their demeanor, we grew closer, supporting each other. Intimidation was their weapon of choice, pounding us with rapid questions and not listening to anything we said.

I realized I had major ego problems. I didn't want to sound stupid. If I couldn't grasp all the terminology thrown at me, I'd just agreed. I was embarrassed, because I wasn't smart enough to understand. I blamed myself for my poor communication skills because I couldn't think fast on my feet. If doctors didn't understand the seriousness of our concerns, I felt I wasn't a good communicator. We honestly felt we were on our own because we didn't take their advice and put Robin in an institution.

We slowly gained confidence in ourselves and began to take back control. After all, we were paying for these visits. We collaborated and started

---

20 www.gentlerevolution.com.
21 www.theautismcentre.co.uk.

making lists of questions we wanted answered. We asked for explanations of things we didn't understand. We did not encourage conversation about the weather; rather we focused on the good in Robin's evaluations instead of just the negative comments. Any progress was powerful to us.

Robin's disability was a shock to us, but equally shocking was the fact that our insurance wouldn't help pay for Robin's schooling, evaluations, testing, or therapies. Thus, financial decisions often took precedence over Robin's needs. We quickly realized that there was a lot I could do to offset expenses at home. I worked with teachers and therapists to develop realistic home plans.

Mental Health Needs

There were many decisions and realizations during Robin's early years. In addition to the girls' and Robin's issues, it was important that we took care of our own mental health. Bob and I became stronger and more focused. Self-help classes were becoming popular, and we took several. Two significant books for us were *I'm OK You're OK*, by Thomas Harris (Avon Books, an imprint of Harper Collins Publishers, 1973) and *Born to Win*, by Muriel James (Addison-Wesley, 1973).

Bob and I knew our mental health was paramount for our family. His sister Jeanne and her husband, Steve, were newlyweds and babysat all three girls several times while Bob and I had weekend getaways. Bob took annual leave from work one week a year and was Mr. Mom. One year I went to Florida and sat on a friend's lanai drinking coffee for a whole week. Another year, Mom and I drove to Arkansas to see my grandmother. In those early years, my vacations and his business travel gave us the space we both needed to survive. Our lives had to consist of more than just Robin.

Because of Robin's behavior I couldn't ask friends to babysit. We hired a sitter, Mrs. Lee, to come into our home one day a week so I could help out in the girls' classrooms, go to lunch with a friend, and grocery shop. Because of Bob's overtime and travel, my structure became paramount for our family's survival. I remember after Christmas that year, Bob said, "We have to let Mrs. Lee go until our bills are paid." I'd overspent. I said, "We'll eat beans first. Mrs. Lee isn't going anywhere!" We both knew I was right.

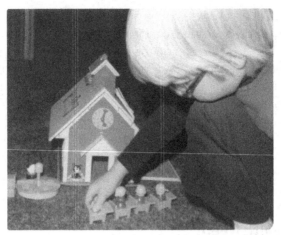

Fig. 11.1. Robin lining up her toys.

I was rooted in the grief of Robin's potential and the grief of our life's circumstances. My guilt wasn't about what caused Robin's disabilities, I couldn't change that. Rather, my guilt was over not doing enough to help her. Whatever I did, it just wasn't enough. My guilt for Pam and Karen revolved around the fact that they no longer were the focus in our family. I definitely experienced all the classic stages of grief: numbness and shock, guilt, anger, depression, acceptance, and forgiveness.

For me, our family's survival took priority. I am a positive person and I felt *acceptance* was easy, which it was. I had to believe in myself and I knew I could make this work. Our family unit changed. I changed. I lost my potential for a career, normalcy of any kind, and the freedom to be me. Reality was *acceptance*. Forgiveness, on the other hand, was a little more difficult. I had to *forgive* myself for not meeting my *own* expectations of myself.

I never slipped into clinical depression. At least I don't think I did. When I became overwhelmed, I'd get a regiment of B-12 shots from my doctor. Vitamin B-12 shots gave me the energy I needed to get back on track. In my opinion, B-12 beats Valium or Prozac any day!

We were very fortunate because Bob loved his job. He was respected and he felt accomplished and fulfilled most of the time. I think this definitely benefited our relationship. His job was demanding and we were thankful he found a career path he loved. We both knew money was important so whatever it took to bring home the money, I was happy.

Raising Our Children

Bob focused more on activities with Pam and Karen while I was focused on Robin. Both girls became interested in horses and Bob and I decided this was a good direction for our family. When the girls realized I was willing to move from our house in the suburbs, and they could have their own horse, they had purpose. Bob, Pam, and Karen spent weekends looking for a small farm. They found land and a builder for a house, and I was "invited" for final approval. Bob and I designed the house with the builder, and Bob and the girls designed the barn they would build.

All three girls, including Robin, put up fencing and built the barn on weekends while our new home was under construction. We borrowed a horse, and we eventually added cows, horses, and chickens—albeit at a slower pace than we expected. Bob was the farmer in the family, not me. The barn and animals were something they did together. Surprisingly, this move actually provided us with more family activities. Our family social life revolved around neighborhood backyard holiday picnics, birthday parties, and volleyball games. Families coordinated activities. For example, for the Fourth of July we made a float with a hay wagon, pulled by a tractor. Harvey dressed as Uncle Sam and the children decorated the wagon. Vaughn roasted a pig, Burt had the fireworks, and we all went on a hay ride, adults and children.

The farming community was a very positive experience for the girls and it kept them busy during their high school years. Robin loved being outdoors (see chapter 12: Robin's Siblings).

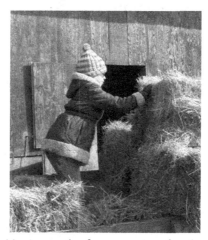

Fig. 11.1. Moving to the farm gave our family purpose.

Many of those years really are a fog today, but I think there are three critical child-rearing decisions that made a significant difference in the outcome of our girls' lives:

1. *Belief system.* Going to church regularly and practicing our faith created a sense of spiritual belonging and community for our girls.
2. *United front.* Bob and I never disagreed in front of the girls. Because of this, they couldn't work us against each other. (Divorced parents can also achieve this same goal.)
3. *Respect.* The girls treated us as their parents, not their peers, and they respected us and our extended families. (If you don't have an extended family, create one.) We respected the girls. The encouragement and acceptance from other adults was important to them. All those Thanksgiving, Christmas, and Easter dinners with grandparents, aunts, uncles and cousins were important, as were neighborhood get togethers. Patriotism and feeling that we were a part of our country was important.

What about money? What about behavior? What about honesty? Everything else, for our family, fell into place when we made faith, family respect, and unity our priorities. In other words, we tried to lead by example.

Our Biggest Decision, Robin's Adulthood

For Pam and Karen, Bob and I had no problem sending them out into the world for college after high school. They were ready and anxious to explore adulthood. For Robin, however, we were not ready to let go. We made a conscious decision to keep supporting her development and see what happens.

We assumed Robin would plateau as she entered adulthood, and we moved into our retirement years when she was twenty-two years old. Although she seldom related to others, her behavior was appropriate in public most of the time. She had attained a minimum language level—although I did most of her talking.

We saw no acceptable solutions on the horizon for her adult life; therefore, she would live with use forever. She was successful because we were successful in managing her boundaries, structure, and consistency. We knew Robin best, and nobody could replace us. Robin and I were the wind beneath each other's wings.

I promised Bob I was done with therapies and schooling. Employment for Robin was always our goal, but the reality was a state-funded adult day program. With Bob's retirement, it was his turn to take the lead when it came to Robin. Now, I wanted the opportunity to have a real job. I would bring home the money to supplement our retirement income.

I never got that salaried job. We slowly realized we were not finished with Robin's development, because she was continuing to progress, even at twenty-four, and again at twenty-eight, thirty, and even thirty-eight years old.

I've been told depression and loneliness are typical in adults with autism and this can often become a greater disability than the autism itself. I definitely agree. Friendships are very difficult and employment opportunities are limited, if they exist at all. And who keeps the same job, routine, or friends for twenty years? As the years have progressed, we have realized we need to keep shaking up Robin's life.

Our first "let go and let God" experience was employment. As Robin's mother, I couldn't believe I was giving her this opportunity. I'd been talking the talk on employment, but now I had to act. From there, things just seemed to happen—friends, driver's license, condominium, second job, and boy friend. Our consistent reinforcement helped her through these learning stages—each was a major step for her.

Admittedly, my biggest anxiety for Robin came when I turned sixty-five. That was the year I got everything in order for my eventual death. Now at seventy, I realize I'm not going anywhere yet. My new goal is eighty-three, and I'm thinking about giving myself an extension!

Today, Bob and I continue to work as a team supporting Robin's independence. We are amazed at how our patience and her determination have merged. There is no way she could have done this alone, and there is no way she's moving back in with us. We love our independent life!

Bob works in the garage on stained glass projects, plays golf, is a toymaker at our church, and is my driver on many volunteer adventures. I've had several part-time jobs, but my expertise is as an advocate for individuals with developmental disabilities and their families. I too keep very busy. My down time includes meeting friends at my Silver Sneaker exercise class at the YMCA and reading.

Bob and I have regrouped many times trying to be objective about Robin's needs. We do not want to overprotect or smother her adulthood. On the other hand, we are very realistic. Outsiders are quick to judge and give their opinions: "Let her make her own mistakes." "You need to live your own life, put her in a group home." "You're overprotecting her." "She has autism, it doesn't matter." "There's nothing wrong with her."

For some people with autism, a group home or assisted living facility is definitely the answer, and someday that might be best for Robin. For now, however, she has shown the ability and desires to have a more independent life.

Confidence and Team Building

Reaching the end of my journey with autism, I silently smile at myself when I think about my favorite children's book, *The Little Engine That Could*. I am that little engine *that could*—I kept chugging and chugging ("I think I can, I think I can"). I love watching tugboats busily moving big ships around a seaport harbor. Tugboats are so small, so strong, and so determined. For larger ships, they work as a team, with other tugboats. That's me! I'm a tugboat. Obviously, I've gained a lot of confidence in myself over the years.

Fortunately, Bob and I both have gained a lot of confidence over the years. It is amazing that even thirty years ago, there were known successes for people with autism. Yes, they weren't published in approved mainstreamed medical journals, but they weren't life-threatening either (i.e., diet and therapies). Many professionals didn't have Robin as their goal; it was all about waiting for the *proven science*. We didn't wait.

Did we turn our back on mainstream medical doctors? Of course not! Robin's progress happened because Bob and I realized that mainstream medicine and alternative medicine, mixed together with common sense, benefited Robin. Did we turn our back on the many autism organizations? Of course not! We needed to understand their agendas—I belong to most of them!

Robin has become a productive adult in spite of her classic autism. Our life was a continual balancing act raising three beautiful children. We survived it. As Robin's parents, we are proud to be walking with her on her autism journey. She can take the bumps and bruises of life. She's her own person. We were told as "long as she's progressing, be thankful."

Well, she's still progressing, and, yes, we are very thankful.

Chapter 12:
Robin's Siblings

Pam and Karen were so excited when Robin was born. They wanted a sister they could hold and love. They didn't understand her behaviors. None of us did. Siblings need such care, husbands too. And so did I.

Pam's personality was much like Bob's—she just fell into the stream of things. Karen, on the other hand, was closer to Robin's age. I often felt she was trying to make up for Robin's disabilities. They grew up fast. Many times, they just learned to stay out of the way. Life was much more serious for them than their peers.

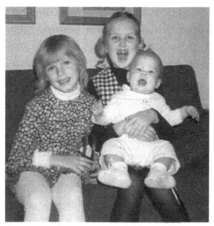

Fig. 12.1. Pam and Karen with Robin.

Pam and Karen were typical girls who took their schoolwork seriously. Outside activities included piano for Pam and ballet and tap lessons for Karen. Later, Karen was a cheerleader for a youth football team, and Pam started horseback riding lessons. Bob and I made it a priority to keep their lives as normal as possible.

Robin was five years old when Pam was in the fifth grade. Pam came home from school one day, crying, and I asked, "What's wrong?" Pam said the teacher was reading a story to the class about Helen Keller, and her classmates were wildly running around during recess hollering "retard" at each other. I talked with the teacher, of course, but I also reread the book.

Helen Keller was blind and deaf, and her teacher, Annie Sullivan, detailed Helen's behaviors—all of which we saw in our own home. Oh, I remember so well dreading the dinner hours.

When Pam was in the tenth grade, the school showed a movie about the danger of taking street drugs and drinking alcohol. The movie's message was that students could prevent birth defects and retardation in their future children if they just stayed away from these temptations. Pam told me about the movie when she got home from school. It was obvious she was very upset because people might think Robin's autism was due to my drug or alcohol use. This absolutely blindsided me. I watched the movie and Pam was right. That is exactly what the movie said!

Both girls graduated from college. Pam chose to graduate college as an occupational therapist (OT). The profession has been very good to her and it has given her an excellent background for raising our grandchildren. Today, Robin gets free OT advice! Karen has a degree in business administration and she was pursuing a second degree in chemistry, before she married and started her own family. Now she's our diet counselor.

The girls care a great deal about Robin's future and we visit often. Both girls have wonderful husbands and both families practice their Christian faith. They have accomplished everything Bob and I ever envisioned for them.

Looking back, my *driving force* was always that each of our children would find happiness in their lives. When Pam and Karen moved out into the world, it was really important to me that they had a life of their own. I did not want them to be responsible for their sister, Robin. As time passed, I had no idea their lives benefited from Robin being the focus of our family all those years.

Pam home schools their three children. I just love it. She has charts everywhere. Leah and Adam play musical instruments and take horseback riding lessons, including horse shows. They have two horses, a barn, and a horse trailer. Pam also takes horseback riding lessons. Adam and Aaron are in the Civil Air Patrol.

Karen's family moved from a mountaintop outside Albuquerque to town several years ago. They are on an organic, gluten-free casein-free (GFCF) diet. She is also home schooling their son. Her stepchildren are all in college and a very important part of her family—the oldest graduates this year.

When Bob and I visit Pam, we get the grandkids. They stay with us at the local Hampton Inn, in one room with two double beds. We play Canasta in the reception area and swim in the pool. They love the free all-you-can-eat breakfast bar. They are teenagers now and will soon find interests that do not involve their grandparents. But for now, they have our undivided attention.

It's a special time for me, and I feel it's important for them, too. Hopefully, they will remember this when they have grandchildren.

Karen's family flies in for a week once a year. Her husband and Robin go neck-deep swimming in the Gulf of Mexico. She loves that. Their seven-year-old son gets to go to the beach every day. He loves that. There are no beaches in New Mexico, and he thinks it's awesome. Grandma has beaches. I also play games with him and give him my undivided attention. Family is full circle.

A Word from Pam

There is no lifelong turmoil or angst from being raised with Robin as my younger sibling. It is a matter of fact. You look at a situation and you learn how you are going to deal with it, then move on to living. You problem solve and work the problem, and you keep doing it until God moves you on to your next challenge.

When I reflect on growing up with Robin, I think of three areas: purposeful play, dietary changes, and determination.

Learning how to play made sense to me even at my young age. Of course, at the age of ten or eleven, I didn't think of it as *purposeful play*, yet the home programs that the therapists sent home taught us how to interact with Robin. Seeing our interactions with her result in a new movement or a new understanding was literally life changing for both of us. As she grew, I became interested in what I was going to do with *my life*. I realized that I wanted to go to college and learn how to help others. I now realize that I became an occupational therapist as a direct result of this *play with a purpose*.

At first, the dietary changes may have seemed a hardship—I really don't remember. What I do remember is the effect one mistake could make: Robin would return to a state of confusion. Even as a child, this consequence was so dire that I really didn't mind our whole family being on the diet. It certainly helped us not let her cheat, because we felt guilty eating something in front of her. It was much better not to have that temptation at all. I do remember grocery shopping with Mom and eating a whole bag of Oreo cookies while shopping (Mom ate them too, it wasn't just me). That way they wouldn't go home. It was fun, and it happened more than once.

Determination and structure were the cornerstones of my life. I always liked that, and even today I am very structured (of course, my family would laugh thinking of my laundry room). Whether it was purposeful play, a structured diet, or just the quiet determination to reach the next milestone in development, I liked knowing what we were doing and why. It was a comforting support during rough times. One story of determination from my earliest years with Robin provides a great example of the marriage needed between structure and determination.

I remember when my parents were trying to get Robin to move from the *little potty* to the big one. She was getting so big herself I'm sure they were getting worried that she soon wouldn't fit on her little one. Yet she would not, or could not, make the switch. It made going places difficult. One day, we were all loaded up in the car. My parents took a huge risk. My dad went upstairs and literally smashed the little potty to bits with his foot while everyone was in the car. We then went to wherever our destination was. Upon our return, we *found* the little potty was broken. How sad, we said. Now Robin was going to have to use the big potty, because her little one was broken. I believe from that time on she did—and there was no emotional turmoil. This was how Robin's thought process worked—a simple cut-and-dry concrete answer to the problem. It was a new way of thinking that helped lay the groundwork for how to approach similar problems in her future.

When my own children were born, it dawned on me that I had never held a *normal* baby. I had held, babysat, and treated countless babies and children with various deficits, but this was a first. No tubes to be careful of, no *soft spots* or open areas—just a baby. Bath time was a breeze. It was wonderful, and, yes, I felt a bit guilty. Then I set out into a new endeavor, to study *normal* development. Until this time, I had only read about *normal* development, never seen it firsthand, so I aspired to learn all I could.

Now as I treat children with *deficits* I realize that so many of the children I see are also experiencing quite *normal* emotions and developmental challenges. And I know what I'm talking about—I now have three teenagers.

A Word from Karen

Being the sister to a sibling with autism certainly doesn't result in a normal childhood, whatever that means. There is no question that my childhood was more serious, more real, more worldly, and more independent than most. However, who would I have become if I were some spoiled kid, driven by my parents' dream of a specific career or completely ignored and left to my own devices.

I definitely didn't understand my peers. Life was more intense for me. I had a friend recently who was an aspiring Olympic gymnast. Due to an injury, she dropped out of the program and returned to high school. She told me she was unable to reintegrate with peers, who were more concerned about the color of eye shadow and cute guys. She had lived away in sports camps away from home and family, living a life of intense discipline. She knew more about how the world operated than most. I have another friend whose father died when he was six years old, after which his mother threw herself into figuring out how to support herself and her son. She went back to college and became a lawyer. His childhood must have been pretty intense, ultimately lacking both parents.

The point is, don't feel guilty about the impact your child with autism has on the family. Every experience has impact. With your guidance, this impact can be good. Try to encourage working together, but allow everyone the private time and activities they need. Just do the best you can, which is all you can do. Allow siblings to be angry. Let them get therapy if they want it. I saw a school counselor, and it helped me talk things out. I also had a favorite uncle I liked to hang out with because he was someone different. But is that so different from any other child?

On the other hand, some research suggests that the first-degree child (the closest sibling—that's me) may have similar difficulties to the child with autism. It is not remarkable to find families with more than one child with autism, with varying levels of severity.

I had a lot of issues growing up. It wasn't until I was in my late twenties that I found out I had a number of learning disorders, including dyslexia. Although I was an honor student in high school, I always felt stupid. The diagnosis I received was that I was "twice special," both learning disabled and gifted. Too bad no one determined that in high school!

In my late thirties, after adopting my beautiful son with my wonderful husband, I decided I was sick of the depression I had. It was ridiculous. I had everything I ever wanted, so why was I sad? I was about to go to a doctor and demand antidepressants when my pastor advised I go see his alternative doctor. Following this visit, my weak immune system was detoxified, debugged, and refortified. This doctor advised me, based on applied kinesiology, that I go on a gluten-free casein-free, soy-free diet. It wasn't until I began to feel better that I came to realize I probably had chronic fatigue syndrome most of my life.

I think my health issues are probably directly related to Robin, whether genetic or environmental. Don't miss this possibility when you are dealing with autism. The siblings in your family may be facing similar obstacles. Of course, don't obsess over the idea, either. Normal growing pains are also to be expected.

My difficulties were very subtle, and I never would have investigated alternative sources if not for the constant search for Robin's *cure*. Because of my parents' relentless search to help Robin, I was willing to try anything to *cure* myself. That is a skill I couldn't have gotten any other way.

Back to growing up with Robin. I remember the rise in intensity in the house whenever there was friction with the school system. I never really understood this, and it took me forever to realize that this household intensity related to stuff going on with Robin. Not knowing was very confusing.

Probably the most significant thing I remember is that I felt it was my job to wake Robin up when she was rocking in bed at night and my job to get her back to sleep without rocking. Perhaps it's these kinds of responsibilities that gave me my work ethic today. There is a good side to every burden. No burdens at all create weak people.

Robin is amazing, but she will always be affected by autism. I am so thankful for my parents' relentless efforts in giving her every opportunity to improve. I come from a long line of strong-willed people. I'm also glad they didn't give up when they were told she was too old to improve.

Nonetheless, the time will come when my parents are no longer with us. One way or the other, either Pam or I will move to live near Robin, or she will come to live near us. Perhaps it will be after Robin retires. That is a normal process for normal people! I know when I told my mom this plan she was not happy. She wanted to be sure Robin could live on her own so that our lives would not be affected. My response was simply that if my other sister, Pam, needed my support, I would want her to come live near me. I would want her to be near family. Robin's case is no different.

I now have a son who has some sensory overload problems. I also have three stepchildren who had an emotionally rough childhood. Over and over again, I see how God provided me experiences in my childhood to help my children recover from theirs. Over and over again, I seek out alternative treatments to help myself and my family. I am able to think *outside the box* to improve our lifestyle. This is directly related to growing up with Robin. I am thankful for the family God chose to place me with.

Chapter 13:
Building Our Plan: A Recipe for Success

The cause of Robin's autism did not matter, we kept telling ourselves—it just didn't matter! Robin was never going to survive in *our world* with her behaviors. She had to change. We began to recognize occasional glimpses of hope in Robin and her fleeting ability to think—we called these *light bulb* moments. We valued these moments as positive growth and we wanted more. We wanted her to be a part of *our world*, and this gave us something to build on. For example, for safety reasons, my discipline of choice was placing Robin in timeout. She spent a lot of time in timeout.

- Robin's sister, Karen, had a friend over to play Barbie dolls. I put Robin's timeout gate across Karen's bedroom doorway so Robin could watch them play. In the past, I'd never used the gate anywhere except at Robin's doorway. Robin ran in circles, because she thought somebody else was in timeout besides her. Now that was smart!
- During a football game the commentator said, "The Redskins will now go into timeout." Robin stopped dead in front of the TV, excited, flapping her hands and staring at the screen. She heard somebody else was going into timeout besides herself. She's been an avid football fan since that day.

Understanding Autism

Many psychologists' evaluations forty years ago were more concerned about whether a person was severely retarded, moderately retarded, or mildly retarded if they appeared to have a mental disability. Most professionals looked at Robin's level of retardation, commenting on her speech, socialization, and behavior as a sidebar. They did not connect all the dots and they usually ended their evaluations with "This child should be retested next year."

By the time Robin was ten her test scores were slipping into the severely retarded range. I read books and attended local conferences, teacher trainings, and community college classes trying to understand her learning style. I looked at everything that might benefit her.

Although autism was suggested to me at an early age, accepting that Robin had autism was a gradual process. She was so different from any other children with developmental disabilities. I finally began reading books specific to autism and joined national autism organizations.

Robin's Unique Needs

When Robin was little her behaviors demanded that—she wanted what she wanted when she wanted it. In her early years, I focused on therapies to help her integrate into the world around her. When Robin was a teenager, we learned to recognize the importance of tailoring everything to her learning style. As an adult, however, change is good, and we've been able to help Robin become responsible and assertive, yet remain in control of her life:

- Carol lives with her parents in Robin's condominium community. Robin has not been good at reciprocal friendships, although she considers Carol one of her best friends. It has taken several years, with my firm prodding and Carol's patience, for Robin to automatically call Carol on her own. They now coordinate rides to social activities, meet for clubhouse events, or go swimming. Carol is an instigator at matchmaking and has successfully encouraged Robin to have a boyfriend.
- Robin told me she wore three heavy coats to work because it was cold. I asked, "Why did you need three coats?" She said, "You told me to layer." I redefined layering and had her purchase some undershirts. I talked about appropriate layering, using examples of some of her clothes. The following Sunday she sat with us in church, took off her coat and smilingly said, "Is this okay?" Her clothes were layered appropriately.

Robin's Unique Gifts

Robin keeps everyone around her on their toes. She's very detailed and I seldom question her accuracy. She has a sense of humor and values her independence. Her quirks are her gifts. She'll never run out of toilet paper or cat food. Other examples:

- Robin's first and best communication with people when she was a child was to catch them with outdated license plates or state inspection stickers. Her language would always be in a scolding tone ("You're bad..." or "You're going to jail"). Recently,

Claire, my neighbor, knocked on the door when Robin was at our house. Robin said to Claire, "Happy birthday." Claire said, "Robin, how did you know it is my birthday?" Robin said, "Your license plate expires on Monday." I was shocked, Robin couldn't have been more appropriate and this shows the tremendous progress in her socialization skills. Claire thanked Robin and renewed her license before it expired.

- After three months as a cashier at Publix, Robin still had her cashier position. I made an appointment with her manager to ask about the rules and regulations of the cash drawer. During the meeting, the manager started flipping back and forth through the shortage notebook and laughed. Robin didn't have a page—meaning she had no errors. *Autism at its finest!*

Seeking Professional Medical Help

Medical safety and interventions are not a *"we against them"* issue—meaning traditional medicine vs. alternative medicine or parents vs. professionals. We should all be on the same team, using medical and educational treatment interventions responsibly to help individuals with autism.

After Robin's pediatrician refused to discuss diet as a possible benefit for her, we realized that most medical doctors have no experience with disabilities. Medical doctors cannot be *all things to all people*. Having said this, I've been surprised how disability programs continue to depend on them to prescribe services. As examples:

- I asked Robin's pediatrician for a prescription for occupational therapy sensory integration (OT/SI) on the advice of a teacher. He said he didn't understand OT/SI, but "Okay, what should I write?" I had to go back to the teacher for the correct wording for him to write the prescription.
- Robin needed her annual prescription for language therapy as an adult. Her local MD would not write the needed prescription. He did not understand the importance of continuing her language therapy to stabilize her autism in adulthood. Fortunately, we have a doctor who has attended the Defeat Autism Now (DAN) conferences, and he wrote the prescription for her.

Medical research, particularly in the past, has focused on medicine—not therapies, vitamins, supplements, or learning styles for autism. Although this is beginning to change, as Robin's parents, we still have problems educating ourselves and finding information to benefit her.

Bob and I have had to be vigilant to ensure we are getting the right information. Many mainstream medical professionals criticize us, often referencing copyrighted published medical studies we did not have access to read. Rather, they expected us to accept an abbreviated summary of the study or the press release version. To make matters worse, television personalities report as if they are medical authorities on autism, promoting the American Medical Association (AMA) or American Academy of Pediatrics (AAP) position, reinforced by the Food and Drug Administration (FDA) and the Centers for Disease Control and Prevention (CDC).

In addition, families of children with autism have become political pawns. Many autism organizations have their own federal and state lobbyists fighting hard for their own personal agendas. Some are trying to dictate approved treatment plans for families along with age and disability limitations. Families have become fundraisers, focusing on research into the causes of autism, not the treatments.

I shiver when I read about intervention programs only for children under the age of five or that a child is too severe to receive help in a specific program—leaving the child rejected and abused by the very system they need, without direction. Thank goodness I didn't listen to professionals when they declared that Robin could not benefit from OT/SI or diet or an education. In her adulthood, my gut instincts led me to the Defeat Autism Now (DAN) protocol. Thank goodness.

It is a very difficult time for families to know which bandwagon to get on. There is no *cookie-cutter* treatment plan for autism. My suggestion is to not let anyone discourage you—educate yourself and keep an open mind. Then invest, pray, and plan.

Negotiating the Networking Maze

Each individual with autism is unique. Robin needed a coordinated program that included family support because she was progressing more at home than at school; therefore, we became her case managers.

Through the years, we did find good medical doctors, psychologists, teachers, and therapists who recognized Robin's development was dependent on our involvement—the parents. Bob usually went with me for evaluations. We valued their time and didn't expect free services. I always went prepared, taking a list of questions with me to all appointments. I made sure I understood what they said, and I listened. It was very important to listen. On the other hand, it was important they listened to us and respected what we had to say. After all, we knew Robin best.

Finding the right professionals for us was usually a gut feeling, an instinct. We did not flip from professional to professional. When we made our decision, we stuck with that plan to give it time to benefit Robin.

We have definitely made poor decisions and mistakes over the years, but we also learned from them. Bob and I accepted this as part of *doing business*. We did not allow these mistakes to discourage us; rather we just changed course. Below are some of the lessons we learned:

- If appropriate, expect goals and objectives to be a direct result of appropriate testing, not guesswork.
- Make sure your therapists are *qualified* professionals and up to date on new coordinated technologies and treatment plans for autism.
- Expect a home program to complement the purchased therapy or program for reinforcement.
- Be very concerned if a professional claims they have all the answers for your child. They should know the benefits of other therapies and make appropriate recommendations.
- Professionals are not your best friend. Regardless where their paycheck comes from, they are paid to help your child.
- Do not encourage professionals to waste time talking about the weather or your new shoes if the appointment is about your child, not your mental health.
- Burn no bridges with professionals. The autism community is very small and it is amazing how we returned to previous teachers, therapists, and doctors over the years.

Currently, there are as many *good* therapists as there are *bad* therapists. The same thing applies to doctors, schools, and intervention programs. Yes, many are respected and certified, but they will see autism as an endless financial *well* to draw from, devising a plan of care that best benefits them financially rather than benefits the patient. It is important that families stay involved.

Making Treatment Decisions

Everything I learned to help Robin came from support groups and working with other parents—everything. This included treatments outside mainstream medicine. Once we identified these, we were persistent in finding the right professionals to help us (See appendix A: How to Start an Autism Treatment Plan). This is what benefited Robin:

- *Therapies:* Psychological counseling, occupational therapy sensory integration, and speech-language therapy. There was no *sound scientific evidence* that these therapies were beneficial for autism, yet they were the foundation for Robin's independence.
- *Diet:* For Robin, food definitely controlled her behavior. She was on the Feingold diet for twelve years, then off for twelve years, and she has been on the gluten-free casein-free (GFCF) diet for ten years. Diet gave Robin the vision to see her future. It was exciting to watch her develop from a child into an independent young lady.
- *Ophthalmologist vs. optometrists:* We had major difficulty correcting Robin's crossed eyes (strabismus) because of her mental and behavior delays. Local ophthalmologists said eye surgery was too risky. After extensive research, we finally found an ophthalmologist who performed two eye surgeries (at four and seven years old) on Robin. Several years later, I made an appointment with an optometrist who specialized in special education students' vision problems. She prescribed prisms in Robin's glasses and said I needed to reteach Robin everything, because she wasn't properly processing visual information. In addition, she recommended art therapy, which Robin received.
- *Dramamine:* A friend gave me a book by Harold Levinson, MD, *The Solution to the Riddle—Dyslexia* (Springer-Verlag, 1980). He was an associate professor of psychiatry at NY University Medical Center. According to Dr. Levinson, he focuses on calming the base of the brain, which is in fluid, to allow the upper brain to learn. This also has a direct relationship to inner ear disorders. He used over-the-counter Dramamine (a motion sickness medicine), vitamins, and prescription drugs.

  When Dr. Levinson interviewed Robin, he looked at me and said, "What are you doing here?" I told him I'd read his book, and I thought he could help Robin. He agreed to try and help her. After returning home, I started Robin on the vitamins and worked with him by phone, because the Dramamine was not helping her. He said it was too strong. He finally found her tolerance level with Marezine at 0.25 mg a day. Dr. Levinson has written seven other books and he is still a practicing MD.[22]

- *Multi-sensory study:* Shortly after we moved to Florida, Robin was invited to participate in a multi-sensory learning research study through some of the families I'd met in my networking. It involved self-help tapes and accelerated learning. I knew Robin benefited from this approach, so without hesitation we moved to the study site for six weeks. She loved it. Admittedly, she had my undivided attention during this time, but it was clear that she had benefited tremendously from the study. It reminded me of our home schooling days and it helped me realize the importance of productive structure and boundaries for her daily living. Sadly, the study did not receive additional funding and it was halted. When we returned home, Robin got her first job, bagging groceries.

- *Auditory Integration Training (AIT):* A parent suggested Robin complete the ten-day AIT therapy. This appealed to me because Robin's evaluations always noted that her auditory system was very weak. Robin completed the program. Using a headset, AIT exposes the person receiving therapy to specific sounds to rehabilitate and balance the auditory system, including distortion.[23]

- *Chiropractic therapy:* Robin has seen several chiropractors throughout her life. Her anxiousness and slow mental processing were always a concern to me. These sessions seemed to help her during times of crisis. In addition to body adjustments, some would do *muscle testing* designed to target her need for specific vitamins and supplements. This technique is commonly referred to as *applied kinesiology,* and it requires extensive training to be done properly. Robin held each bottle of vitamins, one at a time across her chest. She held the other arm straight out to her side and her chiropractor gently but firmly pushed down on that arm. Depending on the strength in her arm, he would say, "She needs this one" or "She doesn't need this one."

22   www.levinsonmedical.com.
23   www.aitinstitute.org.

Managing Family Life

Robin demanded the full attention of our household. We were very thankful she was our third child. We didn't know any better, and we treated her like our other girls as much as possible. We are very fortunate because we stuck together and accepted our family's circumstances. Because of Bob's travel, the girls and I became a team. They grew up fast. Whatever they wanted, it had to wait until I finished with Robin. I know it wasn't easy for them. All we can say today is that we did the best we could!

When Robin started the Feingold diet, we saw significant changes in her behaviors (see chapter 2: Diet, Vitamins, and Supplements). The girls saw them too. Looking back, I believe the diet actually helped our family become closer. Pam and Karen became educated on proper nutrition and good eating habits. We all read labels. Bob specialized in pronouncing all the chemical ingredients on food labels. The girls realized switching to correct products, eliminating packaged foods, with preservatives designed to increase shelf life, was a healthier lifestyle for our family. Keep in mind this was in 1975, when not many people were reading labels.

As a family, we've made it! There is no doubt the main reason, however, is because I was able to be a stay-at-home mom.

Chapter 14:
Finding Support Groups

Everyone knows the importance of support groups or going to counseling for alcoholism, weight gain, or even divorce. We were no different. Bob and I needed supports to raise a disabled child.

Identifying with other families through support groups helped me avoid costly mistakes. I learned which professionals to avoid, where to buy the best products, and ways to love, teach, and raise Robin. I learned to trust my instincts and be a driving force for change, however small.

I found I did best with short-term projects, and I was careful to only tackle one thing at a time. Our family was my priority. I learned to focus my efforts on areas where I could make a difference, not unproductive projects and meetings. I didn't limit myself to just one disability arena, and I never used my volunteering as my own personal spotlight. For some reason, I always knew when it was time to move on.

When Robin attended Muriel Humphrey School for Retarded Children (at two years of age), they embraced the whole family, not just the child. The school was sponsored by the Association for Retarded Children (ARC) and the ARC *expected* family involvement.

I was assigned an *infant stimulation coach*. The coach came to our home every couple of weeks and gave me ideas to coordinate Robin's school and home program. The ARC held monthly support group meetings for mothers while our children were in school. These mothers became my new best friends. We organized fundraisers for the school and attended county supervisor and school board meetings representing all our children's needs.

Moving Past My First Support Group

Robin was four years old when I read *Why Your Child Is Hyperactive*, by Benjamin Feingold. Following this, I saw a notice in our local newspaper about a Feingold diet support group forming in our area. I was very confused about substituting foods and I needed help. The group grew rapidly, and I learned a lot from them. I was a Feingold diet counselor in my area for twelve years. As a diet counselor for other families, we were able to share success stories and it kept me motivated to help Robin.

I attended my next support group when I had trouble understanding the new federal special education law, *PL 94-142: Education of All Handicapped Children Act.* The Parent Educational Advocacy Training Center (PEATC), based in northern Virginia, held training classes for parents, and I became involved in their organization. This training was very helpful, as it showed me what I should expect from the school system. As part of my continuing education, I volunteered for the group, writing and presenting training programs for other families.

Robin wasn't fitting into any disability category. To cover all her disability bases, I need my feet in both arenas—ARC and ACLD (Association for Children with Learning Disabilities). I became a member of our county's public school Special Education Advisory Committee and later the Chapter 10 Mental Health and Mental Retardation Services Board. As parents, we worked with professionals and politicians. We knew what our children needed. I was definitely part of a team. Examples of how I grew to help Robin:

- *Understanding how a child learns:* Northern Virginia Community College (NOVA) developed a mandated curriculum for public school special education teachers' aides. Parents were invited to attend. I learned to recognize the developmental learning stages for children with disabilities. This course helped me understand the brain and that our children can learn.
- *Phonics reading program:* Public school teachers invited the ACLD to participate in a forty-hour workshop called *The Writing Road to Reading,* by Romalda Bishop Spalding (QUILL, Harper Resource, an imprint of Harper Collins Publishers, 1957-2003). Teachers wanted our support for teaching this method to students in special education. I took the course. Little did I know this class would be my foundation for home schooling in the future.
- *Gymnastic classes:* Parents started MAGIC classes—Mastering Adaptive Gymnastics in Children. *PL 93-112: Rehabilitation Act of 1973,* section 504, required public funds to include people with disabilities. The county recreation department welcomed our assistance in finding students and a teacher.

Robin was eleven years old when NBC television aired *"Vaccine Roulette."* It was a show about reactions following a DPT shot. I listened as Marge Grant talked about her son Scotty. I was dumbfounded, because I believed Robin's doctors when they told me vaccines did not cause disabilities. Parents responded to the show and I joined the new-formed parent organization. I felt I needed to learn all I could about vaccine reactions.

Including Robin in Support Groups

When we decided I was going to home school Robin, Bob and I dropped all our extracurricular activities, placing our total focus on Robin. We knew it was going to take our full commitment as we tried to integrate her into typical community activities. Our local newspaper had announcements for new majorette classes and a new 4-H club (see chapter 6: Socialization and Self-Image). These activities became our networking and support groups, and Bob, Robin, and I became active in both for seven years.

While home schooling, I began to focus on learning about autism. I became a member of the Autism Research Institute (ARI), the only newsletter I read cover to cover when it arrived in the mail. Founder Bernard Rimland, PhD, has done an incredible job educating families on autism research and sharing hope for the future. He gave the full interpretations of medical studies, not just the press-release version. ARI started the Defeat Autism Now (DAN) conferences over fifteen years ago for parents and professionals.

After moving to Florida, a newsletter came in the mail for a one-day conference in Orlando, Florida, called The Biological Treatments of Autism and Pervasive Developmental Disorder (PDD). From reading my ARI newsletters, I was familiar with many of the speakers' names—Andrew Wakefield, MD, Bernard Rimland, PhD, Jeff Bradstreet, MD, William Shaw, PhD, and Lisa Lewis, PhD. I told Bob I wanted to attend this conference as my Mother's Day present. The focus was Leaky Gut Syndrome, vitamins, supplements, and the gluten-free casein-free (GFCF) diet.

I had been convinced for years that Robin's chemical sensitivity was a major disability for her. I also felt her diet issues were more involved than the Feingold diet but I could never connect the dots. I requested a scholarship for Robin, and we went to the conference as a family. Robin was now twenty-eight years old, and the conference changed her life.

We were so used to doing things as a family that Robin naturally blended into the support group arena with us as an adult (see chapter 6: Socialization and Self-Image). We focused on things that included her so that she could learn and benefit—which she did.

Chapter 15:
Managing Financial Costs

When Robin was a child, we paid all the bills, including private schooling, evaluations, and therapies. We didn't have a choice. Thankfully, *United Way* did offset some of her expenses when she attended Muriel Humphrey School for Retarded Children. When Robin had her complete evaluation at ten years old, everything became much more expensive. Private evaluations, schools, and therapies were beyond our financial means, but we never considered not doing them. We took out a second mortgage on our home, knowing that we could only afford private school for one year. Our parents had passed away during this time and left us some money. Bob worked overtime. We spent it all on Robin.

Our medical insurance did not pay for evaluations, therapies, or schooling. Researching our insurance policy, we realized it would pay for psychological counseling. I need a guide, I needed a support system to help Robin; thus, Robin had an educational psychologist for over five years. This was a tremendous help and kept us on our path to help Robin.

Robin didn't receive Supplemental Security Income (SSI) when she was a child because of SSI resource and income limits. Prior to age eighteen, the income and resources of the parents were all that count—that is why Robin and many children with disabilities do not qualify for SSI when they are children. When a child turns eighteen, Social Security law considers them an adult, and only their own income and resources count, not the parents' income.

It is important to know what type of benefit your child receives because the rules are different for each program and type of benefit. Social Security Disability Insurance (SSDI), Social Security Disabled Adult Child, and Supplemental Security Income (SSI) are the most common benefits your child may be receiving. They may receive more than one type of benefit; for example, SSDI and SSI. In this case, a different set of rules will apply to each benefit.

There are also rules that allow you to continue the medical insurance (Medicaid or Medicare) even if the cash benefit stops because of work and earnings. If you receive SSI and your medical insurance is Medicaid, the 1619b continuation rule may allow you to continue receiving Medicaid, assuming you are working and earning enough to stop the SSI check (you should find out what the 1619b rule and income threshold is for your state as part of the work planning). If you receive SSDI or Disabled Adult Child benefits and your medical insurance is Medicare; there are rules that allow you to continue to receive Medicare, although you may have to pay a premium to keep the insurance at some point.

Seeking Supplemental Security Income for Adults with Autism

When Robin turned eighteen years old, I headed to the Social Security office to apply for Supplemental Security Income (SSI) for adults with disabilities. They denied Robin SSI. I didn't realize I needed to be more prepared with medical records and other evidence. I thought her disabilities were obvious. I now know that I should have appealed that first denial.

A diagnosis does not insure eligibility; it's the degree of the limitations. Eligibility is determined based on medical records and other evidence. If Social Security denies benefits, you have the right to appeal their decision.

After arriving in Florida and Robin wasn't employable, I returned to the Social Security office determined to be successful this time. She was twenty-three years old and this time they approved her for SSI. With this approval, she now had SSI benefits, which also included Medicaid health insurance.

Most parents of individuals with autism or developmental disabilities depend on their SSI check to help pay the living expenses for their *adult child* who will live with them indefinitely. Parents support this concept because their sole priority is to *protect their child* until they die. Actually, SSI is a good deal for our government, because it's cost effective.

- Supplemental Security Income: approximately $4,000–$8,000 a year
- Group Home or Assisted Living Facility: approximately $60,000 a year
- Jail: approximately $65,000 a year
- Institution: approximately $120,000 a year

Keeping our adult child at home and on SSI may seem like a win-win situation, but this ignores the big picture. Where are our *employment goals*, and how are we making our children *a part of the community*? Where are the rights and choices of a person with a disability? Where is the dignity?

Securing Employment and Social Security Disability Insurance

I never let go of my vision for Robin to become employed. When she got her first job at Publix bagging groceries, she still received SSI. However, for each dollar she earned, Social Security deducted about fifty cents from her SSI check.

Making her own money was a new and exciting thing for Robin. In addition to household expenses, she was now able to take martial arts and piano lessons. As time went on, I went back to the Social Security office, only to learn she now had enough employment *quarters* to qualify for Social Security Disability Insurance (SSDI). Her SSDI benefit was high enough to stop her SSI. Robin's SSDI made her eligible for Medicare and allowed realistic support. Also, Robin continued to qualify for Medicaid under the Medicaid waiver available in our state, Florida. She was set for life, I thought.

Under current rules, the SSDI check is all or nothing. If Robin works and her income falls *under* the SSDI income limits, she will continue to receive her full check. If she works and her income is *over* the income limits, her check will eventually stop unless she qualifies, plans, and utilizes other work incentive options available.

I became very familiar with the rules and regulations of SSDI. Although the check was the same each month, I had to carefully calculate every month's gross income limit and watch out for weeks with five paydays. I trusted no one else with this responsibility. I found that many professionals not working in the Social Security field can easily lead parents astray, suggesting that they understand SSI and SSDI when they do not. It is important to understand there are several income limits. Fortunately, all this is explained in the Social Security *Red Book*.

Social Security Red Book

A Summary Guide to Employment Support
for Individuals with Disabilities under the Social Security Disability Insurance
and Supplemental Security Income Programs

The current edition of the Social Security Red Book can be found at http://www.socialsecurity.gov keyword "Red Book" or call: 1-800-772-1213 and ask for a copy. This is a *must have* reference.

Subsidy and Special Conditions

Robin could have easily lived within the SSDI income limits while living with us in our home. However, when she moved into her own condominium, she needed more income to be truly self-supporting. I learned to work within the Social Security rules. Robin receives Social Security Disability Insurance (SSDI). The income level that determines when the SSDI cash benefit ends is called Substantial Gainful Activity (SGA). In 2009, the SGA amount was $980. This is a monthly amount and is based on gross income earned in a month (before taxes). There are rules that can reduce the amount of the income that Social Security counts when determining SGA. These rules are Subsidy, Special Condition, and Impairment Related Work Expenses (IRWE).

Robin qualified for a *subsidy* because she did not work at the same pace as other employees, did not have equal responsibilities, or needed more support and supervision than other employees in the same position. For Publix, even though she is an excellent employee with high ratings, she does not scan the groceries at their desired speed and needs assistance with some transactions. At the YMCA, Robin does not have as much responsibility as the other receptionists. She is still learning the position.

These job supports are considered a subsidy. Subsidy is usually stated as a percentage. So, based on the supports, it may be determined the employer is providing a 25 percent subsidy; in this case, only 75 percent of the income would be counted when determining SGA. A subsidy is support provided by the employer. Special Condition support is provided by a third party, such as third-party job coach, and should be considered by Social Security when determining if a person is working at the SGA level.

Becoming Financially Self-sustaining: A Trial Run

As time went on, we needed to decide whether Robin could work and earn enough to replace her SSDI with the goal of working her way off benefits—or if she could only work part time with the goal of working part time and keeping her SSDI.

Robin had too much spare time on her hands working part time. As an independent adult, she needed employment to occupy her time, not state-paid companions or her parents. If she was going to be a part of her community, she needed to develop friendships at her workplace. For this, she needed to work more hours. True independence for Robin means financial independence. This includes the possibility of being independent from SSDI.

We wanted to test Robin's ability to work more hours without giving up her SSDI. So how can we make this happen?

After doing my homework, I found out that Social Security has incentives and rules that allow individuals to test their ability to work. I attended five seminars, hosted by different organizations, trying to understand the Social Security work incentives system, because I could not afford to jeopardize Robin's benefits. The more I learned, the more confused I became. The Advocacy Center for Persons with Disabilities, Inc. (AC) in Florida came to my rescue. Victor Panoff gave me his business card, which read, Protection and Advocacy for Beneficiaries of Social Security (PABSS). I didn't realize that Social Security has free advocacy support for people with disabilities in every state.[24]

It was a scary step, but we were ready to see if Robin could work at a level that would make her independent of Social Security. To have any chance of reaching a goal of financial independence, Robin needed some support to help her reach that goal.

Plan to Achieve Self Support

I heard about the Plan to Achieve Self Support (PASS) in the seminars I attended about Social Security work incentives, but I found it all very confusing. The Florida AC helped us understand how Robin could use PASS and actually helped us with the paperwork. (In your state, if the protection and advocacy center does not help with the PASS paperwork, there should be another organization or agency that will.)

PASS is an SSI work incentive. Robin did not receive SSI anymore, but we were told that people who receive SSDI and have a work goal that is expected to earn enough to stop the SSDI check may be able to get SSI through the PASS. With a PASS, Social Security is able to pay the person SSI in order to pay their living expenses, while they use their other income (such as SSDI or wages) to pay for the things they need to be successful in their PASS work goal. For individuals who do not receive SSI already, the work goal must be expected to result in Substantial Gainful Activity (SGA), which is the income level that would stop the SSDI.

The PASS must include a plan with the steps necessary to reach the work goal. The PASS must also list the expenses needed to reach the work goal. Social Security has people specially trained to process the PASS. You can

---

24   www.socialsecurity.gov, keyword: Protection and Advocacy

find the contact information for the PASS expert for your area on the Social Security's Web site.

For Robin, PASS helped with the cost of her supplements and therapy. We were able to provide information to support that these expenses were necessary for her to be successful in her work goal. PASS also helped with the expense of buying her first car. With her own transportation, Robin would be able to work more hours because she would not be dependent on getting rides from family members. Public transportation is not an option in our area.

Robin's PASS has ended, and she has not worked her way off Social Security yet, but this is still something we hope will happen someday soon.

Dividing the Financial Responsibilities

Robin handles her personal checking account, pays all her bills, and balances her statements. She does most of this online through her bank's Web site. I monitor her spending. In my opinion, abusing her benefits isn't a choice or option for her, and she takes her responsibility very seriously.

I'm Robin's Social Security representative payee. I'm responsible for all the Social Security bookkeeping necessary to comply with their program. Although this is confusing to Robin, she's aware that this money is helping her to become more financial independent in the future.

Managing Social Security certainly is not for the timid or insecure; however, if Robin is going to be financially independent, she needs this support. The federal government is leading the way for individuals with disabilities, including autism, to be self-determined and to lead a more independent life. As Robin's advocate, I have learned to work with and trust the Social Security programs that benefit her. I had to find money to keep her out of jail or an institution. Employment was her key, and Social Security benefits her answer.

It's all in the *SSA Red Book*.

Appendix A:
How to Start an Autism Treatment Plan

Starting an autism treatment plan can be overwhelming, as it can be difficult to accept that your child might have autism. Many families feel tested and become frustrated. They try to correct their child's issues themselves through harsh discipline, with little understanding of autism. Reality is that the parents must change—both Mom and Dad! There is no quick fix! Changes include acceptance, attitude, discipline, quality time, commitment, finances, and a genuine willingness to help your child integrate into the world around them.

Instead of trying to control your child with psychotropic drugs, or showing your anger and frustration with discipline that isn't working, why not take a different, perhaps better, approach. Based on my experience as a parent, here are some steps you can take in creating a plan:

1. *Diet*: As a start, assume your child is chemically sensitive, because this is the easiest thing you can do. Start the gluten-free casein-free (GFCF) diet. If you see no changes with the GFCF diet, add the Feingold diet or other suspected allergy foods. Do not dismiss diet as a behavior trigger for your child.
    a. Keep a daily journal of food and behaviors. Separate times of day (morning, afternoon, evening) or daily routine (getting ready for school, meal time, free time, bedtime).
    b. Review your journal every two days, looking for positive changes. Look for specific things, even a moment's change.
        i. Wasn't angry getting ready for bed
        ii. Sat still at the table for a moment
        iii. Showed interest in something, rather than wandering from one activity to another or fixating
2. *Immune system*: Find a doctor who is familiar with the DAN protocol for diet, vitamins and supplements. Autism success must include identifying leaky gut syndrome, cell repair, and balancing the immune system. If your child is not processing

nutrients properly, it will take longer and be more difficult to benefit from therapies. This is too important to experiment with on your own.

3. *Finances*: Budget a yearly amount to address your child's autism in the professional community ($3,000 is a good place to start). If you do this, monthly therapy expenses or evaluation costs will not seem so traumatic.

   a. Check your insurance policies to see what is available.
   b. Research state programs for assistance with autism.
   c. If possible, set up a tax-free medical account with your employer.
   d. If grandparents or other relatives see your true commitment in helping your child, and the true financial limitations, perhaps they will help financially.

4. *Evaluations and networking:*

   a. Do not rely on friends or relatives who do not understand autism for support. Network with other parents who are successful with their child. They can help you find good doctors, therapies, programs, etc.
   b. If your child's in school, a private evaluation can often give you suggestions the school system cannot give you, because they only recommend what they provide.
   c. Do not allow anyone to predict a negative future for your child.
   d. For some children, medication must be considered; however, weigh the benefits carefully. Many medications can dull a child's intelligence and personality. In addition, they are usually not a solution because they continually need readjustment.

5. *Positive behavior modification.* Consistency, structure, and motivation are very difficult, but mandatory, for improving behavior. I had a psychologist for support, but it was my speech-language therapist who helped me with the day-to-day consistency and structure for positive change.

   a. For positive behavior, parents need to present a united front to their child. Do not allow your child to pull parents against each other. (Even divorced parents can do this.)
   b. Slow down and enjoy your child. Give your child the *processing* time needed to respond to the world around them.

    c. Recognize and compliment your child on positive things they have done. Charting with stickers is an excellent tool. To stabilize positive behaviors, chart things they already do that are right. This helps both of you notice the good things instead of just the bad. Pick your battles carefully and *do not* use positive activities (social events) to punish your child.

    d. Do not talk *at* your child but *with* your child. Have conversation. Let your child *into* your world. Do things together. Walk side by side when going somewhere. Take turns side by side—both doing the same thing—like working in the kitchen. Become a team. For Dad, clean the yard side by side or take out the trash together.

    e. If possible, discourage compulsive behaviors and encourage other areas of interests. This can be very challenging, but sometimes compulsive behaviors encourage the autism behaviors to survive rather that the person with autism to be a part of the world around them.

6. *Therapies*: All therapies should be evaluated by a *professional* in that specific field—occupational therapy sensory integration, speech or language therapy, etc. Parents need to research therapists and make sure they specialize in autism and are up to date with technology. There are many exciting complementary programs available today. Demand home programs and support.

7. *Self-esteem*: It is important individuals with autism feel good about themselves. Make sure you're not expecting more from your child than what's realistic or age appropriate. Research your community for mainstreamed socialization or start something yourself. Find activities with boundaries. Martial arts are often a good place to start. Be creative and stick with it. Try to find activities with immediate rewards. Jumping from activity to activity can be detrimental to your goals.

Diet and supplements, financial commitment, positive behavior modification, self-image goals, professional support, and networking all build on each other. For our daughter, changes to her diet along with positive behavior modification made our household joyful again. Therapies, socialization, and home schooling allowed her self-image to grow and stabilize. Continued biomedical interventions and language therapy in adulthood gave her independence.

She needed it all!

Appendix B: References

Organizations

Autism Research Institute (ARI)
Defeat Autism Now (DAN)
4182 Adams Ave.
San Diego, CA 92116
866-366-3361
www.autism.com

National Autism Association
1330 West Schatz Lane
Nixa, MO 65714
877-622-2884
www.nationalautismassociation.org

Unlocking Autism
PO Box 208
Tyrone, GA 30290
866-366-3361
www.unlockingautism.org

Autism One
1816 West Houston Ave.
Fullerton, CA 92833
714-680-0792
www.autismone.org

Autism Society (AS)
4340 East-West Hwy, Suite 350
Bethesda, MD 20814
800-3AUTISM
www.autism-society.org

Talk about Curing Autism (TACA)
3070 Bristol St., Suite 340
Costa Mesa, CA 92626
949-640-4401
www.tacanow.org

Autism Speaks
2 Park Avenue, 11th floor
New York, NY 10016
212-252-8584
www.autismspeaks.com

National Vaccine Information Center (NVIC)
407 Church St., Suite H
Vienna, VA 22180
703-938-0342
www.nvic.org

Parent Educational Advocacy Training Center
100 N. Washington St., Suite 234
Falls Church, VA 22046
703-923-0010
www.peatc.org

Center for Self-Determination
35425 Michigan Ave. West
Wayne, MI 48184
734-722-7092
www.self-determination.com

Feingold Association of the United States
37 Shell Rd., 2nd Floor
Rocky Point, NY 11778
800-321-3287
www.feingold.org

Celiac Disease Foundation
13251 Ventura Blvd. #1
Studio City, CA 91604
818-990-2354
www.celiac.org

Celiac Spruce Association
PO Box 31700
Omaha, NE 68131
877-272-4272
www.csaceliacs.org

National 4-H Headquarters
Youth Development Cooperative Extension Service
410 8th St, 5th Floor
Washington, DC 20004
202-274-7115
www.4-H.org

Social Security Administration
Office of Disability and Income Security Program
www.socialsecurity.gov (Keywords "Red Book" *or* "Protection and Advocacy")

Reference Books

Chemical Sensitivity and Diet

Barrie Silberberg. *The Autism and ADHD Diet*. Naperville, IL: Sourcebooks, Inc., 2009.

Julie Matthews. *Nourishing Hope for Autism*. San Francisco, CA: Healthful Living Media, 2008.

Karyn Seroussi and Lisa Lewis, PhD. *The Encyclopedia of Dietary Interventions for the Treatment of Autism and Related Disorders*. Pennington, NJ: Sarpsborg Press, 2008.

Lisa Lewis, PhD. *Special Diets for Special Kids Two*. Arlington, TX: Future Horizons, Inc., 2001.

Benjamin Feingold, MD. *Why Your Child Is Hyperactive*. New York: Random House, 1975-1985.

Occupational Therapy Sensory Integration

A. Jean Ayres, PhD. *Sensory Integration and the Child*. Los Angeles, CA: Western Psychological Services, 1979-2005.

Lindsey Biel, MA, OTR/L, and Nancy Peske. *Raising a Sensory Smart Child: The Definitive Handbook for Helping Your Child with Sensory Processing Issues*. New York: Penguin Group, 2009.

Carol Stock Kranowitz, MA. *The Out-of-Sync Child Has Fun*. New York: Penguin Group, 2003.

Ellen Notbohm and Veronica Zysk. *1001 Great Ideas for Teaching and Raising Children with Autism Spectrum Disorders*. Arlington, TX: Future Horizons, Inc., 2004.

Terri Mauro. *The Everything Parent's Guide to Sensory Integration Disorder*. Avon, MA: Adams Media, 2006.

Education, Behavior, Social, and Language

LorRainne Jones, PhD. *The Source for Expressive Language Delay*. East Moline, IL: Linguisystems, Inc., 2003.

Winifred Anderson, Cherie Takemoto, Stephen Chitwood, Deidre Hayden. *Negotiating the Special Education Maze—A Guide for Parents and Teachers*. Bethesda MD: Woodbine House, 1979-2008.

Romalda Bishop Spalding. *The Writing Road to Reading*. New York: QUILL Harper Resource, an imprint of Harper Collins Publishers, 1957-2003.
Nancy M. Hall. *Explode the Code*. Cambridge, MA: Educators Publishing Services, 1984-2005.

Other

Bryan Jepson, MD, with Jane Johnson. *Change the Course of Autism: A Scientific Approach for Parents and Physicians*. Boulder, CO: Sentien Publications, 2007.
Harold Levinson, MD. *The Solution to the Riddle—Dyslexia*. Los Angeles, CA: Springer-Verlag Publisher, 1980.
Jenny McCarthy. *Louder than Words*. New York: Dutton, published by Penguin Group, 2007.
Kathy Hoopmann. *All Cats Have Asperger Syndrome*. Philadelphia, PA: Jessica Kingsley Publishers, 2006.
Barry Neil Kaufman. *Son Rise: A Miracle of Love*. New York: Harper & Row, 1976.
Thomas A. Harris, MD. *I'm OK You're OK*. New York: Avon Books, an imprint of Harper Collins Publisher, 1973.
Muriel James. *Born to Win*. Reading, MA: Addison-Wesley Publishing Co., Inc., 1973.

Web Sites

Diet

- Nourishing Hope, www.nourishinghope.com
- Feingold Association of the United States, www.feingold.org
- Autism Network for Dietary Intervention (ANDI), www.autismndi.com
- GFCF Recipes, www.gfcfrecipes.com
- GFCF Diet, www.gfcfdiet.com
- My Gluten Facts, www.myglutenfacts.com

Parent-based Therapy Programs

- DIR/Floortime model, www.floortime.org
- Hanen, More than Words, www.hanen.org
- Relationship Development Intervention (RDI), www.rdiconnect.com
- Rhythmic Entrainment Intervention (REI), www.reiinstitute.com
- Rethink Autism, www.rethinkautism.com

Therapy-based Programs

- Scientific Learning Fast ForWord, www.scilearn.com
- Interactive Metronome, www.interactivemetronome.com

Other

- Schafer Autism Report, www.sarnet.org
- Age of Autism, www.ageofautism.com
- Autism Hangout, www.autismhangout.com
- Harold Levinson, MD, *The Levinson Medical Center for Learning Disabilities*, www.levinsonmedical.com
- Calvert Home School, www.calvertschool.org
- *Tennessee Microboards* (Guardianship alternative), www.tnmicroboards.org
- Auditory Integration Training (AIT), www.aitinstitute.org

- Glen J. Doman, *The Institutes for the Achievement of Human Potential*, www.gentlerevolution.com
- Carl Delacato, *The Autism Centre*, www.theautismcentre.co.uk

Index